ETHICAL COUNSELLING:
A WORKBOOK FOR NURSES

ETHICAL COUNSELLING: A WORKBOOK FOR NURSES

Philip Burnard, PhD, MSc, RMN, RGN, DipN, Cert Ed, RNT

READER IN NURSING STUDIES,
UNIVERSITY OF WALES COLLEGE OF MEDICINE,
HEATH PARK, CARDIFF

Kevin Kendrick, MSc, BA(Hons), Dip Soc Admin, Cert Ethics and Theol, FETC, Cert Ed, RGN, EN(G), OTN, Post Grad Cert Adv Nurs Prac

ASSISTANT DIRECTOR OF TEACHING AND LEARNING,
SCHOOL OF HEALTH CARE STUDIES,
UNIVERSITY OF LEEDS

ARNOLD

A member of the Hodder Headline Group
LONDON • SYDNEY • AUCKLAND

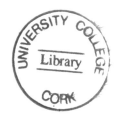

First published in Great Britain in 1998
by Arnold, a member of the Hodder Headline Group,
338 Euston Road, London NW1 3BH

http://www.arnoldpublishers.com

Whilst the advice and information in this book are believed to be true and
accurate at the time of going to press, neither the authors nor the publisher
can accept any legal responsibility or liability for any errors or omissions
that may be made.

British Library Cataloguing in Publication Data
A catalogue record for this book is available from the British Library

ISBN 0 340 60274 0

1 2 3 4 5 6 7 8 9 10

Publisher: Clare Parker
Production Editor: Liz Gooster
Production Controller: Sarah Kett

Composition in 9/11pt Palatino by Phoenix Photosetting, Chatham, Kent
Printed and bound in Great Britain by The Bath Press, Bath

CONTENTS

INTRODUCTION

If you really want to help somebody, first of all you must find him where he is and start there. This is the secret of caring. If you cannot do that, it is only an illusion, if you think you can help another human being. Helping somebody implies your understanding more than he does, but first of all you must understand what he understands. If you cannot do that, your understanding will be of no avail. All true caring starts with humiliation. The helper must be humble in his attitude towards the person he wants to help. He must understand that helping is not dominating, but serving. Caring implies patience as well as acceptance of not being right and of not understanding what the other person understands.

Kierkegaard, 1859

This book is all about the process of caring for, talking to and listening to people. On the face of it, these latter two activities seem to be relatively simple processes. However, they both involve decisions about what we *do* when we talk and listen. This book, then, is about using counselling ethically and about counselling itself. As we shall see, the question of ethics enters into almost every aspect of counselling. But then, so does it enter into almost every aspect of nursing. To practice as a nurse is to practice in an ethical manner. This is as true of counselling as it is of nursing. Also, Kierkegaard, in 1859, seemed to sum up most of the things that anyone in nursing who wants to counsel needs to bear in mind.

What is in the book?

This book asks you to take an active part in the learning process. It is a workbook. You are asked to read through sections of the chapter and then to ask yourself a variety of questions about each passage. The aim, overall, is to get you to question *yourself* – you and your values.

Chapter 1 considers the question 'What is counselling?'. It will help you to decide, for yourself, what counselling is and what it is not. Chapter 2 is about ethics and about the ways in which we choose what is right and wrong. Again, these turn out to be difficult questions and ones that you are invited to consider for yourself.

Chapter 3 identifies ways in which counselling can be used in nursing. It is not suggested that every nurse wants or needs to be a counsellor. But every nurse, at some point, uses *counselling skills*. There is a difference and it is one of the things discussed in Chapter 3. Chapter 4 is about planning counselling.

The next two chapters concentrate on counselling skills themselves. Again, you will be asked to reflect on your own skills and performance with other people – particularly with patients – to enhance your own skill levels. Chapter 7 tackles the thorny issue of whether you can or should use counselling skills in everyday life, with friends, families and colleagues. Is counselling reserved for people we label 'patients' or can everyone benefit from it?

Chapters 8–10 focus on personal development and then on coping with potentially difficult situations in counselling. Chapter 10 deals exclusively with some of the ethical issues that frequently face practitioners when dealing with dying people and their loved ones. We have devoted a whole chapter to this issue because it is a subject that health professionals often cite as a cause of anxiety. Chapter 11 offers you the opportunity to debate and further reflect on a variety of issues about counselling as a whole.

Who is the book for?

This book is for any nurse who wants to learn more about her or his relationship with patients. In the last few years we have seen how important it is that nurses become *reflective practitioners* and that they learn to think and reflect as they work. It is hoped that this book will help in that process.

The book is for clinical nurses and nurse educators (who may want to use some of the activities as part of an interpersonal skills course). It is also for managers and researchers who may gain some ideas for new projects, both management and research.

How do I use this book?

The point of this book is that it is *interactive*. Do not just read through it. Do the activities and answer the questions as you go. In the end, of course, no one can *tell* you how best to use a book. Broadly speaking, these activities will ask you to consider case studies and dialogues that take you to the heart of this book's purpose – to help you to *use counselling skills ethically*. Our intention, in writing it, was to invite readers to be critical of what they read, to be critical of what they think and feel, and to review their own practice. We feel that this will not happen, if all you do is read the 'informative' parts of the text.

The other point that needs to be made is that the book can be used *alongside* other texts. As you work through the book, you will find references and pointers to other books and papers to read. Again, we hope that you will seek out these other works and use them together with this one.

Nursing and caring are intrinsically linked to counselling and ethics; we hope that this book helps you to explore the challenges involved with caring for people in your professional life.

Philip Burnard
Cardiff
Kevin Kendrick
Ilkley, West Yorkshire
June 1998

1 WHAT IS COUNSELLING?

CHAPTER AIMS

- **To enable you to identify the particular features of counselling**
- **To reflect on your own ideas about counselling**
- **To distinguish between counselling and psychotherapy**
- **To identify ways in which counselling is or is not appropriate in nursing**

Introduction

Counselling has been widely recommended as a nursing activity. If we are to discuss the pros and cons of using counselling in nursing, we must first identify what sort of activity it is.

First, it is important to distinguish between *counselling*, on the one hand, and *counselling skills*, on the other. Counselling may be thought of as the activity that people called counsellors engage in. If you are a counsellor, then it seems likely that your main occupation is counselling. Those counsellors use a range of skills that can be referred to as *counselling skills*. There is a wide range of such skills, ranging from simple listening to quite complex, interpretative interventions.

Now while all counsellors use counselling skills (although they will vary in the types of skills they use according to the beliefs they have about how best to help people), it is not only counsellors that can use such skills. We may not all be counsellors but we can still use counselling skills to help people. On the other hand, the equation does not necessarily work the other way round; just because we use counselling skills does not mean that we are counsellors.

This is an important distinction. It is similar to a point that may be made about painting. Various people may use paint brushes and paints for various purposes. Not all of them, though, would claim to be artists. So it is with counselling. While counselling skills have wide application, only counsellors do 'counselling'.

In what sort of situations might nurses use counselling skills? Nursing is such a *sociable* profession – in the sense that it involves working closely with and for other people – that it may be harder to find instances of when counselling skills would *not* be useful. Consider the following list of situations in which such skills might be used and then add your own:

- on home and community visits
- on admission to wards and clinics
- prior to surgery
- when explaining or interpreting what other health professionals have said
- when talking to other staff, colleagues and health professionals
- when talking to relatives
- when sitting quietly with a patient, talking about his or her problems, life situation, feelings or views.

Definitions

Counselling has been defined in various ways. Fifty years ago, the term would probably have been equated with 'advice giving' and this connotation has lingered on. Many people, when asked to say what they think counselling is come up with the idea of giving other people advice. Sometimes, of course, counselling involves just that. At other times, however, *it involves much more*.

Before you read any further, jot down your own definition of counselling. Try to make it as comprehensive as possible.

Ways of approaching a definition of counselling

There are various ways of thinking about what counselling might be. First, we might define it in terms of the skills involved. Thus, we might define counselling like this:

> Counselling is a means of using a range of listening and other skills to help other people work through problems.

On the other hand, we might define it in terms of expected outcomes. A definition of this sort might look like this:

> Counselling is a process that enables people to make life choices and to change their behaviour in ways that they choose for themselves.

Yet another way of defining counselling is in terms of the overall process involved. This sort of definition might be as follows:

> Counselling is a method of helping another person to talk through emotional and life problems in an understanding atmosphere.

Another way of devising a definition is by attempting to tease out the distinctive features of one thing by comparing it with another.

> Counselling is a process usually (but not always) carried out by people called counsellors. A distinction can be made between 'doing counselling' and 'using counselling skills'. While counsellors usually counsel, a much wider range of people may use counselling skills. In this sense, counselling covers the whole process of sitting down with another person, on a regular basis, to work through that person's problems. Counselling skills, however, is a blanket term for a range of interpersonal skills which includes, at least, listening, responding, helping and information giving.

Notice that no one definition can suit all given situations. What definitions do, however, is to help us think about what we are doing and why we are doing it. The sort of definitions cited above are examples of *stipulative* definitions. In each case, they are an expression of one person's view of what counselling is and how that person is using the term at the time. Compare the above definitions with your own and see the ways in which they are similar or dissimilar.

ACTIVITY BOX 1.1

- Carefully read again the above passages.
- To what degree do you feel that the distinction that has been made between 'counselling' and 'counselling skills' is an important one?
- Do you feel that nurses should, as a general rule, have training in 'counselling' or in 'counselling skills'?
- Should certain types of nurses be trained as counsellors? If so, which ones and in which disciplines?

Formal definitions

It is useful to see how other people have defined counselling in the literature. It has, after all, been written about extensively. Noonan (1983) offered a definition that reflects an historical view of the activity but, oddly, noted, too, that it was a 'popular activity'.

> Counselling has its beginnings, both historically as an emerging discipline and daily as a popular activity, in many different professions. It fills the gap between psychotherapy and friendship, and it has become a recognised extension of the work of almost everyone whose business touches upon the personal, social, occupational, medical, educational and spiritual aspects of people.

Aptekar (1955), on the other hand, saw it as a 'private activity' that did not, necessarily, need to be a professional one.

> Counselling can be carried out privately, and without the need to call on agency resources ... all that is required is a person who has a problem and one who is willing to share that problem and bring to bear upon it whatever skills he may have, so that a solution may be reached.

Writing from the point of view of counselling children, Crompton (1992) identified a range of specific foci as a means of defining counselling.

> [Counselling is] help, through the development of a professional relationship, to recognise and manage problems and difficulties connected with and/or stimulated by a range of factors including environment (for example, school), event (for example, bereavement), individual development (for example, sexual), relationship (for example, with parents), movement (for example, within care, between divorced parents), behaviour (for example, offending), and to assist with growth and development in all aspects of the individual person – cognitive, emotional, physical and spiritual.

Meanwhile, Jones (1994) took a more obviously 'humanistic' approach to counselling when defining it as a process leading to personal growth and responsibility.

> An enabling process, designed to help an individual come to terms with his life and grow to greater maturity through learning to take responsibility and to make decisions for himself (Jones 1984).

Mallon (1987) highlights the variety of forms of counselling and, from an educational point of view, defined it thus:

> Counselling happens in many settings, at many times and in many different ways. It is not restricted to private rooms where a confident, fully trained counsellor receives those who wish to be helped. Rather, in most educational settings, a somewhat harried adult searched for a quiet space in which to snatch some time for a distressed child or parent to talk. The contact is often brief, unplanned and unsatisfactory for all concerned, though in many instances it is the best that is available at the time.

Breese (1983) noted the *time* factor involved in counselling.

> [Counselling is] offering a chance to talk freely and openly, individually or in a group in a non-authoritarian atmosphere, on a regular (normally weekly) basis, within a structure of time and place where people have the opportunity a) to be heard and understood; b) to see things from the point of view of others; and ... d) to gain greater understanding of themselves and others.

Reber (1985) took a general, open and fairly versatile approach to definition and suggested that counselling involved many of the processes found in education itself.

> A generic term that is used to cover the several processes of interviewing, testing, guiding, advising, etc., designed to help an individual solve problems, plan for the future etc.

Elsewhere, one of the authors (Burnard 1994) has focused a definition on the need for counselling to involve not only talking but also the need for action.

> The process of counselling is the means by which one person helps another to clarify his or her life situation and to decide further lines of *action*.

This definition is probably a little *too* broad in its remit but it is hoped that it conveys the idea that, in the end, counselling must be more than just *talking*. Something must be achieved by counselling and that achievement can nearly always be stated in terms of behavioural change – or 'action'.

Rowe (1990) offered a slightly ironic view of counselling and suggested one way in which counselling might differ from psychotherapy.

> If people feel that psychotherapy is too pretentious a word to apply to what they do, they describe what they do as counselling.

This highlights a problem that often arises in the literature (and in discussions) about the differences between counselling and psychotherapy. As we will see, other writers have tried to tease out the distinctions between them.

Other commentators have recently been more scathing about the rise in interest in counselling. Dalrymple (1996) writes as follows:

> each age has superstitions of its own. For example, we believe in counselling. Whether we are assailed by debt or diabetes, gambling or gastritis, hypocrisy or hypochondriasis, we believe that counselling will set us free. ... Counselling is the Valium of this era.

The British Association for Counselling (1989) seemed to want to cover all possible aspects of counselling in their definition and, again, offered a broadly humanistic definition.

[Counselling is] the skilled and principled use of a relationship to facilitate self-knowledge, emotional acceptance and growth, and the optimal development of personal resources. The overall aim is to provide the opportunity to work towards living more satisfyingly and resourcefully. Counselling … may be concerned with development issues, addressing and resolving personal insights and knowledge, working through feelings of inner conflict or improving relationships with others.

Not all of the meanings of the words in the BAC definition are self-evident and, in some ways, you have to know something about counselling in order to understand the definition. For instance, the BAC suggest that counselling involves the 'principled use of a relationship to facilitate self-knowledge, emotional acceptance and growth'. It is not clear, though, what might be understood by terms such as 'self-knowledge', 'emotional acceptance' and 'growth'. Nor, later in the definition, will it be clear to everyone what is meant by 'working through feelings'.

The approach taken by Nelson-Jones (1995) illustrated that, unsurprisingly (as a writer on the topic), he had considered a wide range of aspects of the usage of the term.

The term 'counselling' is used in a number of ways. For instance, counselling may be viewed: as a special kind of *helping relationship*; as a *repertoire of interventions*; as a *psychological process*; or in terms of its *goals*, or the *people who counsel*, or its *relationship to psychotherapy*.

Nelson-Jones, perhaps, offers the most exhaustive of definitions and the definition with the broadest scope. It is interesting to review these definitions and to note that some of them define counselling in term of the *aims* of counselling and some in terms of what counsellors *do*, and some attempt to summarise the features that comprise the counselling relationship.

Meanwhile, Hopson (1981) identified the main functions of counselling patients as being able to help them to:

- enter into a relationship where they feel accepted and understood and are therefore prepared to talk openly about their problems
- achieve an increased understanding of their situation
- discuss alternative courses of action

- make a decision about what to do
- develop specific action plans
- do, with support, what has to be done
- where necessary, adjust to a situation that is unlikely to change.

All of these definitions can be compared and contrasted with definitions of psychotherapy – something with which counselling is often confused:

In the most inclusive sense [psychotherapy is] the use of absolutely any technique or procedure that has palliative or curative effects upon any mental, emotional or behavioural disorder. In this general sense the term is neutral with regard to the theory that may underlie it, the actual procedures and techniques entailed or the form and duration of the treatment. There may, however, be legal and professional issues involved in the actual practice of what is called psychotherapy, and … the term is properly used only when it is carried out by someone with recognised training and using accepted techniques. (Rebor 1985)

[Psychotherapy is] the systematic use of a relationship between therapist and patient – as opposed to pharmacological or social methods – to produce changes in cognition, feelings or behaviour. (Holmes and Lindley 1991)

Dryden, Charles-Edwards and Woolfe summarise the differences that are sometimes said to exist between counselling and psychotherapy. They suggest that the following points are made:

- that psychotherapy is concerned with personality change whereas counselling is concerned with helping the individual to utilize his or her own resources;
- that psychotherapy is concerned with people who are in some sense 'neurotic' or psychologically disturbed, whereas counselling is concerned with people who are basically emotionally healthy but who are confronted by a temporary life problem or issue;
- that whereas the focus of methodology for the psychotherapist is the nature of transference between therapist and client, the counsellor is less concerned with this relationship than with helping the client to clarify the issues and develop strategies of management by the counsellor's deployment of a specific set of relatively restricted skills;

- that the psychotherapist is concerned with the inner world of the client as opposed to the counsellor's focus on helping the client to resolve external issues which are generating problems;
- that the work of the psychotherapist is based on psychoanalytical theory, whereas the counsellor's work is inspired by humanistic approaches;
- that psychotherapists tend to work in medical settings, whereas counsellors tend to work in non-medical environments. Thus, the former work with patients and the latter with clients;
- that counselling tends to be a shorter-term process than psychotherapy, and vice versa (Dryden *et al.* 1989).

ACTIVITY BOX 1.2

- Once more read through the points made by Dryden *et al.* and see to what degree you agree or disagree with their views. For instance, is counselling usually a 'shorter-term process than psychotherapy'?

In the end, the distinctions between counselling and psychotherapy become rather 'grey'. It seems likely that many people will see counselling as something that anyone can take part in. On the other hand, psychotherapy is more often associated with the world of medicine and, to a lesser degree, with psychiatry as a branch of medicine. That distinction, however, is not nearly as clear as it would seem as psychotherapy is generally available to anyone who wishes to have it (although rarely available under the National Health Service). Nor are the specific regulations clear regarding the training of those who counsel and those who do psychotherapy. At this point, suffice to say that, for the purposes of this book, it seems to the authors more likely that nurses will feel more comfortable with the idea of their doing counselling and less so with the idea of their doing psychotherapy, unless, of course, they have had specific training in a particular type of psychotherapy.

The whole of this debate does, however, raise the ethical issue of whether or not *all* counsellors and psychotherapists should be regulated. That is to say, whether or not they should be required to be on a register and be able to demonstrate that they have received a formal training and have been in practice for a set number of hours prior to registra-

tion. At the time of writing, however, no such regulation is in place. You would do well to consider this issue and to determine, for yourself, the *degree* to which you engage in counselling people as part of your nursing work. While it seems reasonable to expect that all nurses would offer support and information to patients who are admitted for routine surgery, it may be less reasonable to expect all nurses to be able to offer the required amount of support for someone who is undergoing an acute psychotic breakdown. On the other hand, and to complicate the issue slightly, all nurses in training now have mental health training to at least a minimal degree. The question remains an open one as to when any given nurse is 'experienced enough' to practice as an 'in-depth' counsellor. Perhaps, until regulation comes into force, the suggestion must be that all nurses are self-regulating. This means that each of us, as nurses, should be prepared only to work within the limits of his or her experience and to recognise when it is time for him or her to 'refer on' a particular patient or client.

The question of when to refer on is an important ethical and practical issue in counselling. It is clearly of no value to the client or the nurse if the nurse carries on counselling when she or he is of no therapeutic help to the client. The situation is a difficult one. Having to admit that we are no longer helping is a blow to our self-esteem and to our professional competence. However, we are being much *more* professionally competent if we refer on when the time has come for us to do so. Drawing on the work of Cinebell (1966) and French (1993), it is possible to identify, as follows, the times when a client should be referred on to another professional:

- The client can be helped more effectively by another.
- The client does not respond to the counsellor's offers of help.
- The client's needs take up too much of the would-be counsellor's time.
- The client's needs are best met by established organisations (e.g. Alcoholics Anonymous).
- The client has serious financial problems.
- The client needs medical advice or specialist treatment.
- The client seems to be suffering a mental illness or needs intensive psychotherapy.
- The counsellor is doubtful about the nature of the client's problems.
- The client is severely depressed or suicidal.
- The client's conflicts are of a religious nature and require religious support.

The other remaining issue concerns the degree to which nurses *should* do counselling. Again, we are forced back to the issue of the meanings of words. If we decide that counselling is a particular activity, only to be carried out by very highly trained professionals, then it seems likely that only a very few nurses will operate as counsellors. If, on the other hand, we conceptualise counselling as something that fits comfortably with everyday activity, we might say that all nurses are involved in something of this nature. Although the current emphasis in nursing is on *health*, the fact remains that many nurses, for much of their time, are concerned with caring for the sick. The process of entering into and remaining in the sick role means that people require support and help. It seems reasonable, then, to assume that most nurses will not only be caring for patients in the physical and environmental senses of the term but also in the psychological and, perhaps, spiritual senses. In this case, then, nurses *are* involved in counselling. This point is returned to in Chapter 3.

ACTIVITY BOX 1.3

- As we have seen, counselling is about talking with people and listening to them.
- Consider the following two dialogues and the degree to which the people in them are listening to each other and understanding what the other is trying to convey.

DIALOGUE 1.1

'I worry about what my test results are going to be like.'
'I expect they'll be OK. I wouldn't worry.'
'The doctor seemed happy enough with me.'
'Well, there you are then.'
'Yes, but it doesn't stop you worrying, does it?'
'No. That's natural. Everyone does that. I suppose it doesn't do any good to worry, though. Does it?'
'No. You're right. I just wish I knew a bit more about what was going on.'
'You'll know soon enough. As soon as they have any news, they'll tell you. And I bet it will all work out OK.'
'Do you think so?'
'Yes, of course.'

DIALOGUE 1.2

'I worry about what my test results are going to be like.'
'What, particularly, are you worried about?'
'The results, you know.'
'If the results are not good? That's what's worrying you?'
'Yes. If I've got cancer, really . . .'
'You're worried by the thought of cancer?'
'Yes. Very. I mean, what would I do?'
'What has the doctor said?'
'He's said there's only a very small chance that I have.'
'Did he say anything else?'
'Yes . . . he said he was almost certain it wasn't cancer. Yes, I'm being daft, really. It's better just talking about it, though. Thanks.

QUESTIONS ABOUT THE DIALOGUE

- What were the main differences in the *approach* used in the two examples?
- What do you feel was the 'better' conversation?
- Why?
- How could either of them be improved?

REFLECTIONS

These two examples involve a patient who has undergone diagnostic tests. One possible outcome is that the investigations will reveal cancer. In both examples, the patient is asking questions that invite the nurse to give an informed response; these type of questions are sometimes called 'open-ended' because they demand more than a 'yes/no' answer. The response given by the nurse in each situation is, however, very different.

REFLECTIONS ON DIALOGUE 1.1

In the first dialogue, the nurse gives very 'closed' responses that fail to encourage the patient to explore worrying issues; for example, the nurse says 'I expect they'll be OK. I wouldn't worry' as a response to the patient's perfectly warranted worries about test results. By responding in this way, the nurse closes any real opportunity to engage with the patient. This pattern is mirrored throughout the whole of their dialogue.

One of the biggest challenges faced by human beings is dealing with the unknown. This is something that confronts us from our earliest days of development; for example, the main reason that many children are frightened of the dark is because it masks their known world. If we cannot see what is around us, it becomes very difficult to engage with and understand it. Such notions stay with us throughout life. Horror writers and cinematographers have capitalised fully on this – it is often the suspense of not knowing, rather than 'blood and gore', that gives a movie its Gothic splendour and the ability to frighten.

However, fact is always more frightening than fantasy; thus, when the patient expresses fears about test results it links to the most virulent of fears – that of the real unknown. When this also concerns the possibility of a life-threatening illness, the patient is confronted by trauma of the unknown and facing mortality – a 'double whammy' of immense proportions.

Dealing with the unknown is also closely linked to another primal theme – the need to feel in control. This is an essential human want – the ability to exercise governance over matters relating to the way we live life; this is often called 'autonomy' by ethicists. In an excellent book on informed consent, Faulder (1985) offers an interpretation of autonomy that can be directly applied to nursing practice: 'the individual's freedom to decide her or his goals and to act according to these goals'. However, the idea of absolute autonomy is something of a myth – nobody can be fully independent and self-governing.

Consider the term 'autonomous nurse'; it is facile to think of an individual's practice as something which is free of constraints. As nurses, we have to work within a framework which is influenced by a Code of Professional Conduct (UKCC 1992), the organisational milieu and the needs of patients – thus, total autonomy is not reconcilable with the limitations of the real world. These themes are reflected by Henry and Pashley (1990), who state that:

> full autonomy is an ideal notion and we can only approximate to it. It is obvious that, in reality, some situations, states and circumstances will diminish a person's autonomy (such as, the ability to control his or her actions, or both) through being restricted in some way, e.g. illness, psychological impairment, physical or mental disability.

Despite the cogent borders and limitations that

Henry and Pashley place upon autonomy, it remains a key feature of practice that nurses should work with patients to lift barriers that prevent the expression of governance. Occasionally, patients may make it known that they wish to take no part in decision making and want to leave it entirely in the hands of health professionals; commenting on this, Kendrick (1991) states:

> The patient should be given the freedom to say to the nurse that he wishes to surrender any role within the decision making process. This agreement may be temporary or permanent in nature. What must be emphasised here, is that when a patient gives the nurse responsibility for decisions he does not relinquish autonomy, but gives acknowledgement of it.

A central issue arising out of Dialogue 1.1 is that the nurse does not offer the patient freedom to ask for and, just as importantly, receive information that directly relates to vital health issues. Without this information, the patient cannot begin to manage a terrifying situation.

In essence, the patient has asked the nurse for help in exploring palpable fear and anxiety. By giving closed and dismissive responses, the nurse gives the message that this is not feasible. In doing this, the nurse destroys the possibility of a therapeutic relationship, dwarfs trust and denies any willingness to engage with the pragmatics of advocacy. This leaves the patient in a position where:

- Fear of the unknown remains a stifling reality.
- Fear of cancer and death remains unexplored.
- The lack of control remains constant.

It often takes courage to ask for help. The very act of seeking help sometimes gives signals that we are vulnerable; showing this goes against a primal biological instinct that mirrors Darwin's notions about 'survival of the fittest'. It is ingrained in our culture that you cannot be both 'vulnerable' and also one of the 'fittest'. Such themes can often act subliminally to stop patients asking for help. Nursing, however, is intrinsically about helping people who are vulnerable; this should be a positive, nurturing and enabling process that makes a person feel safe about acknowledging vulnerability.

In the first dialogue, the nurse has denied the patient access to these most human themes; not only has any chance of meaningful and therapeutic dialogue been squandered but also trust in other nurses and health professionals may have been irreconcilably damaged. This is a dreadful price to pay for not responding to a patient's cry for help.

Nobody is saying that the nurse in the first dialogue has been deliberately evasive or intended to harm. Contemporary practice takes place in a frantic milieu where demands on nurses and time are very intense. Conversely, it may just have been that the nurse was having a 'bad day' – we all have them – and 'to err is human'. Whatever the reason, most of us will have been in situations similar to this nurse.

The first thing to do when we have mishandled such a delicate dialogue with a patient is to revisit them to try and make amends: a simple 'I'm sorry, I don't think I listened very well to what you said before' is often enough to reopen the door and help a patient to explore their fears. Indeed, the mere act of saying 'sorry' and acknowledging our own shortcomings is often a great leveller and may even help the patient to feel more comfortable with you.

If it is not possible to revisit the patient, then reflecting upon the dialogue and learning for future encounters is a focused and cogent means of improving the skills we bring to such scenarios. Writing about the importance of reflection to nursing practice, Parnell and Kendrick (1995) state:

> Reflecting upon our own experiences is rather like looking in a mirror; it helps individuals to gaze at a scenario and learn from the images it presents. We can never actually go back and live through an occurrence again, but thinking about the events that formed it allows for contemplation and can help contribute to our learning.

What we can certainly say about Dialogue 1.1 is that what the nurse offers falls short of the essential themes in counselling – especially listening skills. We will now explore the second dialogue to discover if it offers the patient a more open arena for exploring fears.

REFLECTIONS ON DIALOGUE 1.2

In the second dialogue, the nurse takes a much more open and focused approach to dealing with the patient's queries – open because the replies given encouraged the patient to talk about the exact source of worry and anxiety; focused because, similarly, each reply mirrored the patient's question and helped to confront the real target of fear, that is, whether or not the tests will reveal cancer.

What this dialogue shows is that the nurse 'actively' listened to what the patient was saying and helped put the worry of cancer directly in proportion to what the doctor had already said. This sort of dialogue shows how carefully chosen responses can, in a short space of time, help people to understand their fears and use strategies for coping with them. The fundamental power of listening to others is that it gives people the opportunity to share worrying thoughts, fears, feelings and emotions; as the patient said, 'It's better just talking about it'.

When nurses engage with patients in this way, it enacts an ethical theme that holds particular resonance for nursing practice – respect for persons. This concept is closely linked to autonomy; exploring this further, Faulder (1985) states:

> Deeply embedded in the principle of autonomy is the concept of 'respect for persons', and one of the ways of expressing that respect is always to assume that they wish to exercise their rights unless they indicate otherwise.

This duty to enact the principle of respect for persons is a cogent thread throughout the Code of Professional Conduct (UKCC 1992); Clause 7 holds particular relevance for the interpersonal aspects of the nurse–patient relationship:

> Recognise and respect the uniqueness and dignity of each patient and client, and respond to their need for care, irrespective of their ethnic origin, religious beliefs, personal attributes, the nature of their health problems or any other factor.

Such themes are given a further specific focus towards communication in the document *Guidelines for Professional Practice* (UKCC 1996), which states:

> Communication is an essential part of good practice. The patient or client can only make an informed choice if he or she is given information at every stage of care. You also need to listen to the patient or client. Listening is a vital part of communication. Effective communication relies on all our skills. Building a trusting relationship will greatly improve care and help to reduce anxiety and stress for patients and clients, their families and carers.

The second dialogue shows patient–nurse interaction that clearly fulfils the guidelines offered by both the UKCC documents referred to here.

ACTIVITY BOX 1.4

Think about the issues in this chapter and, in particular, about the business of talking and listening. Then answer the following questions:

- Are you a better 'talker' than 'listener'?
- Can you think of a person whom you would describe as a 'good listener'?
- What sort of person are they?
- What do they *do* when they listen?
- What could you do to improve your own listening skills?
- What sort of person do you like to listen to you?
- Who listens to you best of all?

Conclusion

This chapter has opened the debate about counselling. It has identified various ways of defining counselling and acknowledged that there is no one 'right' way to define it. The chapter has also alluded to a difference between *counselling* as a process undertaken by trained counsellors and *counselling skills* – a range of interpersonal skills that may be used by a range of caring professionals.

What has emerged is that counselling skills are an essential part of the nursing remit. A central feature of this is the ability to listen and respond appropriately when patients are asking questions that reveal anxiety and worry about care-related issues. This process, if handled sensitively, can embellish and enrich the interpersonal relationship between nurse and patient.

We have also discovered that the therapeutic relationship between nurse and patient should reflect the ethical principles of autonomy and respect for persons. Throughout this book we will continue to explore the ethical dimensions of interpersonal skills in the nurse–patient relationship; the importance of ethics to nursing is given particular buoyancy by Tschudin (1993):

> Ethics is not only at the heart of nursing, it is the heart of nursing. Ethics is about what is right and good. Nursing and caring are synonymous, and the way in which care is carried out is ethically decisive. How a patient is addressed, cared for and treated must be right not only by ordinary standards of care, but also by ethical principles.

Having set ethics firmly at the centre of the nursing endeavour, the next chapter will develop this further and consider some ethical theories and their relevance to counselling.

2 THE ETHICS OF COUNSELLING

CHAPTER AIMS

- To consider the nature of *ethics*
- To explore ways in which ethics relates to counselling

Introduction

Ethics is intermingled and woven throughout the whole of this book. The purpose of this chapter, however, is to give a brief overview of some classical ethical theories and apply them to case studies and dialogues that reflect situations where nurses have to use counselling skills. In writing this chapter, it is our hope that the ethical theory we cover will inform the way you engage with and respond to activities, case studies and dialogues throughout the rest of the text. Some of the activities ask you to consider situations that may not fit neatly into a traditional counselling setting but that certainly make demands upon counselling skills. Whenever possible, we have used examples from our own experience or the experiences of people we have worked with (all case studies and dialogues have been disguised and names changed to preserve the anonymity of those involved).

Definitions

Perceptions of ethics are as varied as the morals that inform individual behaviour. Some people see ethics as an abstract subject that belongs firmly in the ivory towers of academia; others see it as a subject that parliamentarians manipulate in matters of political controversy. There are elements of truth in both these perspectives; ethics is, however, much more than this.

Unlike many words, the essence of ethics cannot be succinctly reflected in a single definition. Building on this, Sparkes (1991: 206) questions the usefulness of dictionaries and argues that the best which can be offered for ethics is an interpretation *not* a definition; this is given as 'The philosophical study of moral conduct and reasoning'.

Sparkes' interpretation gives direction and focus to the essential purpose of ethics. In essence, it is concerned with the way in which reason can clarify situations that have a moral dimension. This last point gives a rationale for placing ethics at the centre of the nursing equation, since the focus of that profession is steeped with issues that demand ethical enquiry and a moral response.

ACTIVITY BOX 2.1

- Write down three ways in which you think ethics is used in your everyday life (choose either professional or personal examples).

Making difficult decisions is part of the fabric of everyday life. This may be deciding where to go on a group outing – How can you choose a place that will make all members of the group equally happy? It may be to do with money – Should you put money in a charity box that would help starving children when you really fancy a chocolate bar and have insufficient money to do both? It could be deciding whether or not to take a bit longer on your morning break: you are really tired and it has been 9 days since your last day off – your ward, however, is short-staffed.

What this exercise shows is that ethics informs the way we live our lives. Ethics is a feature of interaction with other human beings. When people meet, in whatever capacity, it is almost certain that issues will arise that have an ethical dimension. This may not be a deliberate process and the people involved may not realise that they are engaged with ethics; indeed, if we are honest, the important dilemmas we face in everyday life are usually characterised by an uncomfortable feeling in the pit of the stomach and a wish that someone would wave a magic wand and make the situation right. Of course, magic wands are the things of fairy tales while ethics is well and truly rooted in the real world.

Ethics, then, is about questions of right and wrong and about what might be good and what might be bad. There are various ways of thinking about questions of right and wrong and some of them are described here. The following section also shows how the various approaches link to nursing and counselling.

The 'greatest happiness' principle

The philosopher John Stuart Mill, drawing on the political philosophy of Jeremy Bentham, argued that what was 'right' was that which caused the greatest happiness for the greatest number. A right action, then, is one that causes the most people to be happy as a result. Not surprisingly, there are problems with this approach. For example, it is not such a good principle if you happen to fall into minority categories. It might also be an excuse or an encouragement to marginalise people. Those who are not in the 'majority' – and these might include, for example, the mentally ill, gay people, single-parent families, and so on – might have decisions made against them through the application of this principle.

On the other hand, we might argue that the principle allows individuals, in counselling, to make decisions about their lives. The 'right' decision, in this case, would be one that the client makes that effects the greatest amount of happiness for the greatest number of people in his or her life. The downside of this is that the decision may be one that the client does not want to make. This is an important feature of utilitarian thinking – self-sacrifice must be accepted if it promotes the happiness of the majority.

The 'greatest happiness' principle applied to counselling

The greatest happiness principle might be used in counselling to help patients to decide on what they should or could do. For example, helping a patient to identify the likely implications of decisions for various members of their family and their friends may help them to decide on what it is they want to do.

A major problem with utilitarian method is that, while it states that happiness should be promoted, it fails to define what happiness actually is. This can have major implications in a counselling scenario. Even if a patient decides that a certain course of action will lead to happiness on an individual basis and for everyone else concerned (the majority), there is no guarantee that this will actually happen. For example, one of the authors (K.K.) once nursed a man who smoked 30 cigarettes a day and drank 5 pints of beer a night. This man was in hospital because of pronounced hypertension. During conversation, the man revealed that he was worried about dying of a heart attack and wanted to stop smoking and drinking for himself and his family (he was married with two young children). A plan was devised, with the man's full involvement, to gradually make lifestyle changes.

The man left hospital with his blood pressure controlled and a firm resolve to stick to the lifestyle changes. From a utilitarian perspective, the stage was very well set: a course of action had been chosen that should promote happiness for all concerned – the ideal utilitarian scenario. Unfortunately, the man died 3 months later from a stroke. This highlights a central failing of utilitarianism: there is no guarantee that a given course of action will lead to happiness for the majority – it certainly did not in the example we have given here. Thus, trying to decide what will promote happiness before the fact is not without its failings; crystal ball gazing is a poor basis for moral deliberation.

Kantian theory

Immanuel Kant, an eighteenth-century philosopher, asserted that respect for people is the primary test of one's duties. The points of his approach to ethics might be summarised as follows:

1. All people must be respected *as* people. They must be treated as 'subjects' and not as 'objects'.
2. A person must respect himself or herself as being human. A person should not treat himself or herself as an object.
3. People must be treated as *means* and not as *ends*. That is to say that *how* we deal with people is as important as the *outcome* of what we do.

A shorthand way of denoting Kantian ethics is often illustrated by the phrase that 'we should treat others as we would, ourselves, want to be treated'. This is sometimes called the *golden rule* in ethical philosophy. It also has implications for counselling. Clearly, if counselling is concerned with 'treating' people in a broad sense, then two things arise out of this: first, counselling is an *ethical* activity and, second, when counselling, we should treat the client only in such a way as we would approve of for ourselves.

APPLYING KANT'S THEORY TO PRACTICE

A glaring problem with duty-based approaches to morality (deontology), and Kantian ethics, in particular, is that they tend to portray certain principles as absolute, universal and all-encompassing. This can have definite limitations when viewed against the often fraught and traumatic nature of nursing.

ACTIVITY BOX 2.2

■ Read the following case study which is adapted from a real experience; all names used are fictitious.

It is coming to the end of a late shift on a medical ward and Paul, a staff nurse, is updating patient care plans. One of these patients is Jane Smith, a 32-year-old woman suffering from a fractured arm, three broken ribs and numerous facial abrasions and bruising. These injuries are allegedly the result of an assault by her husband; the police are involved and are currently trying to locate this man's whereabouts. Out of concern for Mrs Smith's safety, a police officer has been placed at the entrance to the Nightingale ward, just in case her husband should try and reach her. Although shocked, Mrs Smith is going to press charges as she has 'had enough of the beatings'.

Paul realises that the television is on in the day room and goes to switch it off as nobody is in there. After turning the TV off, Paul is suddenly aware of another presence in the room; he turns urgently to be faced by an aggressive and alarming man who demands 'You've got me missus, Jane Smith. Now, I want you to be a good boy and tell me where she is'. Paul is terrified, he does not know what to do and is frozen with fear.

■ Write down what you would say to Mr Smith when told: 'You've got me missus, Jane Smith. Now, I want you to be a good boy and tell me where she is'.

REFLECTIONS

Incidents involving aggressive and violent behaviour are confronting nurses with increasing regularity. Although this incident cannot be classified as a classical counselling scenario, Paul certainly has to use very sensitive listening skills and respond sensitively to Mr Smith's aggressive behaviour; in this respect, handling and managing aggressive behaviour makes great demands upon a nurse's counselling skills. Paul has only a second or two to respond to the man's hostile request; if he fails to comply, it may lead to personal injury. If he does disclose Mrs Smith's whereabouts, it may mean putting her in grave danger. There is no absolute moral principle which guarantees the most appropriate way to proceed in this situation.

If Paul firmly believed that the truth should always be told, then he may feel a strong obligation to divulge Mrs Smith's whereabouts (this would strongly reflect the deontological approach of sticking with the rules, irrespective of the consequences). After all, it is not the telling of the truth which may cause harm, but the actions and intent of the husband.

Conversely, Paul may identify more with the themes of utilitarianism, with its emphasis upon actions being morally justified if the result is happiness or pleasure for the majority of people, or limiting the harm which would otherwise affect them.

Applying this to the present dilemma, telling Mr Smith a lie may safeguard the interests of the majority of those involved. For example, Paul may say that Mrs Smith was currently being questioned by the police in another part of the hospital, which may gain just enough time to alert the police officer to Mr Smith's presence. This would benefit Paul, Mrs Smith and the rest of the patients on the ward. Such an approach draws a clear connection between the act of lying and the hope that it will lead to positive consequences. This is fundamentally different to deontology, which would emphasise that telling the truth is inherently good and quite separate from the immoral actions of another person – in this case, Mr Smith.

Of course, the result of either approach may be traumatic. Neither deontology nor utilitarianism can provide a crystal ball and it is impossible to know the results of an action beforehand. Paul has only seconds to make a vital decision – it is a harm-limitation exercise; every option carries risks. However, what this case study reveals is that there may be occasions when a nurse telling a lie can be morally justified. Moreover, it must be remembered that the nurse, irrespective of moral considerations, has a clear duty in law not to make an unauthorised disclosure about confidential information – law and ethics often make uneasy bedfellows.

This section has considered two opposing ethical approaches – Kant's theory and the greatest happiness principle (utilitarianism) – in relation to a volatile and highly charged scenario that makes full demands upon a practitioner's counselling skills. Life is never as simple as always sticking strictly to the rules, as situations sometimes arise where rules have to be 'bent' or even broken; for example, as a general rule it is morally justified to say that nurses should not lie. In the case study, however, Paul may have thought that lying to Mr Smith was the safest way of preventing a dangerous situation from developing into a more harmful scenario.

Equally, to spend life living by the utilitarian principle of the 'greatest happiness' can lead to a rather shallow and hedonistic perspective where the only moral endeavour is to search for pleasure, irrespective of the consequences that this may have for the minority. From this perspective, rules can be wantonly broken if it promotes happiness for the majority.

In the real world, most people live their lives within a sort of moral conglomerate that unites both Kantian and utilitarian perpectives; there are rules that have to be respected and adhered to (in most situations – remember that it is the exception that often proves a rule's worth). Likewise, there is little harm is seeking happiness or pleasure so long as it causes no harm to others.

Appeal to a code of conduct

This section follows on suitably from Kant's advice to adhere strictly to rules, since it deals with the use of codes as a means of providing people with a form of moral framework. Most of us are affected by a range of codes of conduct. Some of us will have particular religious beliefs, and at the centre of most religions is a code of conduct telling believers what is right and wrong in terms of personal and social conduct. The religious person, then, is told what is right and wrong for them by appealing to this code. Sometimes, an interpretation of this code is required to fit this particular set of issues at this particular time. In these cases, it is usual for an elder in the religious organisation to be entrusted with such interpretation.

Nurses have to subscribe to their own Code of Professional Conduct (UKCC 1992). This document identifies a range of 'rights and wrongs' regarding professional behaviour both within the nurse's professional span of duty and in their wider, personal life. Again, this code of conduct will help in enabling nurses to make 'right' decisions about certain things.

There are, of course, problems with codes of conduct. As we have seen, they are usually written in terms of broad principles and require interpretation by a human being. As human beings are usually fallible, it seems likely that the individual who requires advice on right or wrong is left to accept the interpretation of another human being. It is only if this other human being is assumed to have some sort of 'special' ability for discerning the truth of the code in question that we are likely to be completely happy with the outcome of this sort of decision making. In essence, then, codes provide the starting point for discussion, analysis and professional discernment but they are not categorical absolutes. Chadwick and Tadd (1992: 14) pursue this line of enquiry and comment:

> A code of conduct or ethics should perhaps be seen, not as the last word on ethics, but as a stimulus to moral thinking.

Codes provide a 'window' through which professional dilemmas may be viewed. However, merely 'viewing' a dilemma has little impact upon it and further analysis is needed to address all aspects of a difficult situation; ethical analysis can provide the necessary 'tools' to help achieve such an endeavour.

The conscience

Drawing on Freud's idea of the *superego*, it is possible to argue that what is right is that which our conscience 'tells' us is right. According to this principle, we all carry around with us the internalised values of our parents. At an early age, we were all affected by what our parents thought was right and wrong. To a greater or lesser degree (so this argument goes), we continue to be affected by these notions as we grow up. The point, then, is that what is right for us is what our conscience dictates to us. The downside of this principle is that it would appear that we are 'trapped' by our consciences and no allowance is made for our freely choosing a course of action.

Applying the conscience to counselling

This may have less obvious implications for counselling. One application, though, is through inviting the patient to identify what they *feel* they should do. Asked in this way, the question is an invitation to address the conscience. The question remains, however, as to what degree the conscience *should* always be 'listened to'. Many of us carry around with us (from childhood) a great number of 'should nots' and 'must nots' which have long since outlived their usefulness; for example, few adults cling to their parent's command to be in bed by a stated time. Ironically, this is yet another way in which 'conscience' can be used in counselling. The nurse first asks the client what his conscience tells him to do and then asks if this is what he *wants* to do; for example, a nurse may ask a patient, 'What does your conscience tell you about smoking 60 cigarettes a day?' The likelihood is that the patient's conscience will be at odds with what he or she actually wants to do.

Existential ethics

Existentialism is a way of philosophising, usually associated with philosophers such as Kierkegaard and Sartre. The slogan that best sums up existentialism is *existence predates essence*. This takes a little explaining and we can do this though an example that John Paul Sartre used. If we take a paper-knife, we will note that before it came into existence, someone designed it with its function (or its *essence*) in mind. Someone, at some point, said 'What does a

person need in order to open letters easily?' The design led to the existence of the paper-knife. Once in existence, the paper-knife remains a paper-knife for the rest of its existence. We can say about such a knife that its *essence (its design) predated its existence*. For Sartre, in the case of human beings, exactly the opposite is true. We first of all exist, live a little and then *define ourselves*. Thus, our existence comes first and then, as we grow up, we define our essence. We are authors, if you like, of our own essences. This being the case, we are also deciders of what is right and wrong for ourselves. We may like to look to codes of conduct or to other people's opinions of what we should and should not do but, in the end, *we* have to decide what is right and wrong for ourselves. This, then, is the position of existential ethics. There can be no clear set of principles to follow. Each person must decide for himself or herself.

One of the problems with this approach is that it can be extremely disconcerting and uncomfortable. As Sartre says, we choose in anguish. We can never know, beforehand, whether or not the path that we choose towards being right is the correct one or the best one. We always have to act on less than sufficient information. In many ways, though, the client-centred approach to counselling is based on this idea of existential ethics, that is, of the person choosing for himself or herself.

Existentialism applied to counselling

The use of existential ethics in counselling is fairly clear. Here, the nurse helps the client to work out exactly what *he or she* (the client) wants to do and stresses the fact that only the client *can* decide. This must, however, be done tactfully and sensitively. Not everyone can face the idea of being free to choose in this way. Nor does everyone accept the principle that we *are* free. Others would argue for what is called *determinism*. Determinism is the principle that every event (including human, cognitive and affective events) is caused by prior events. That is to say that everything we think and feel is linked to prior experience. Thus, true freedom of thought is a myth. Marx, the political philosopher, took this one stage further and argued that *society* works along determined principles. Thus, the individual is *not* free to choose but, rather, is part of the determined society in which he or she lives. All of these issues raise interesting questions about the nature of counselling.

If people *are* free to choose, then counselling would seem to have a definite place and, more particularly, the client-centred approach would seem to have a place. After all, if it is the client who decides, then it is appropriate that the counsellor helps in that process and does not attempt to detract from it by offering their own opinions and views. If, on the other hand, people are *determined* and have little or no say in what happens to them, then we may be left with the conclusion that counselling is *not* a useful activity. For, if we are truly determined, no amount of *talking* about a situation could change it. One of the authors (P.B.) is reminded of running a client-centred counselling course in a Muslim country. The course went well, but at the end of the week a course participant said to the author 'Why do you bother with this client-centred approach? In the end, Allah will sort it all out one way or the other.'

ETHICS OR MORALITY?

Ethics, then, is the study of what is right or wrong or, perhaps, how we can *consider* what might be right or wrong. In contrast, 'morality' is the living out of ethical codes. People have morals and *study* ethics. In this sense, ethics is the *formal study of morality*. Sometimes, though, the terms are used as synonyms.

In counselling, there are various ethical issues to consider and a short list of them would be as follows:

- Is it *right* to counsel people?
- Should you always have another person's *permission* before you counsel them?
- Should you advise people about what they should and should not do?
- What if a person asks you a direct question about right and wrong?

As may be expected, there are no cut and dried answers to these questions, but they are worthy of debate.

AN ETHICAL CODE FOR NURSES

In thinking about how nurses might act in a counselling relationship, it might be wise to identify what *rights* nurses have. Curtin and Flaherty (1982) offer a useful list of what they called *earned rights*:

- the right to practice nursing in accord with professionally defined standards;
- the right to participate in and to promote the growth and direction of the profession;

- the right to be trusted by members of the public;
- the right to intervene when necessary to protect patients, clients or the public;
- the right to testify authoritatively to the community about the health care needs of people;
- the right to be believed when one is speaking in the area of his/her expertise;
- the right to be respected by those inside and outside the profession for one's knowledge, abilities, experience and contributions;
- the right to be trusted by colleagues;
- the right to give to and to receive from colleagues support, guidance and correction;
- the right to be compensated fairly for services rendered.

Curtin and Flaherty also point out that the rights are also an accurate reflection of the *duties* of nurses. All of this has direct relevance for counselling as a nursing activity. If you read through the list, it becomes evident that in undertaking counselling, within the framework of these rights and duties, various expectations are apparent. For example, as a nurse-counsellor, you have the right and duty to be respected by colleagues. This means, also, that your conduct, as a counsellor, must be beyond question. Read through the list and consider ways in which *you* believe such a list impinges on a nurse's work as a counsellor.

ACTIVITY BOX 2.3

Before you read further, write down as little or as much as you choose in *answer* to these questions. Think carefully about what *principles* are behind your answers.

- Is it right to counsel people?

Much, here, will depend on how counselling is defined. When we ask such a question as this, we need to ask a previous question, 'How are you defining counselling?' If, as we saw in the previous chapter, counselling is viewed merely as a form of talking and listening, then we may argue that this is what everyone does, most of the time. Counselling cannot be ruled out as a 'wrong' activity if it is part of what the average person does with people around him or her. If, on the other hand, we want to mark out counselling as a 'special' activity, involving experts trained in counselling, then we might answer the question by saying that counselling *might* be the right thing to do on two conditions: (1) that the counsellor is trained and (2) the client has *asked* to be counselled.

ACTIVITY BOX 2.3 – *contd*

- Should you always have another person's permission before you counsel them?

This point has been dealt with, to some degree, above. Clearly, if a person is qualified to counsel (and much will depend, as we have seen, on how counselling is defined) and someone asks for counselling, it seems reasonable to offer it. A question, however, hangs over *when* someone is deemed to have asked for counselling, or, put another way, when they have given their permission for another person to counsel them. We might say that if a person begins talking about problems and is obviously keen to get another person's views on those problems, then permission has, covertly, been given. However, there is another circumstance in which things might not be so clear, and this is illustrated in Dialogue 2.1, below.

- Should you advise people about what they should and should not do?

To answer this question, we need to revisit some of the ethical principles identified above. If, for example, we take an existential view of ethics, we might say that we *cannot* advise people about what they should and should not do. On the other hand, if we have strong religious convictions and these are shared by the person we are counselling, we might want to remind them of their obligations under the code of conduct. This applies, too, in nursing situations where a nurse-counsellor may think it appropriate to remind another nurse of their obligations under the Code of Professional Conduct.

- What if a person asks you a direct question about right and wrong?

This is probably the most difficult one of all. The answer seems to be that we have to make *some sort* of response. We might try to dodge the issue by saying something like 'It isn't important what *I* think, it is you that we are talking about.' But this does just that: it dodges the issue. The client may well repeat, 'Yes, but what do you *think*'. Another approach to the question is to say, rather long-windedly, something like 'This is what I would do but I am not suggesting that this is what *you* should do'. One of the authors (P.B.) favours a more direct approach by saying 'In my view, this is what you might think about doing.' The final approach is to explore a range of possibilities with the client and to get the client to *identify* those possibilities.

DIALOGUE 2.1

In this example, the issue is whether or not the nurse is behaving appropriately in inviting the client to talk. The question to answer here is 'Has permission been given for counselling to take place?'

'How are you feeling at the moment?'
'Not too bad, thanks.'
'You look a bit miserable.'
'Do I? I feel OK. I always look a bit grim!'
'There seems to be something bothering you.'
'Well, I've got a few things on my mind.'
'About your family?'
'Not really.'
'About your boyfriend?'
'Well, yes, actually.'
'What's the problem?'

QUESTIONS ABOUT THE DIALOGUE

- What are you feelings about this nurse's approach to the client?
- Should the nurse have pursued this line of questioning?
- What would have been the appropriate way of finishing this conversation?
- How would *you* have handled this if you were the client?

ASSESSMENT ACTIVITY BOX

Think about the issues in this chapter and then answer the following questions:

- Is it right for *you* to counsel people?
- How do you make ethical decisions?
- Should you advise people about aspects of their lives?
- If so, what sorts of aspects?
- Should your religious convictions, if you have them, affect what you do as a nurse?

Conclusion

A central theme of this chapter has been to discover and consider some of the key features of the classical schools of ethical thought. It would be impossible, within the space of a single chapter, to describe how the schools of ethical thinking covered here could be applied to every situation you may meet where counselling skills are used. What we ask is that during the rest of the book you continue to make reference to this chapter; for example, you might ask yourself what a utilitarian or Kantian approach would be in a given case study or dialogue. In this way, the theories that we have touched upon in this chapter will become alive and vibrant to you.

3 COUNSELLING AND THE NURSE

CHAPTER AIMS

- **To explore situations in which nurses might use counselling skills**
- **To examine the limitations of counselling in the nursing role**
- **To begin to explore how nurses might learn counselling skills**
- **To explore issues of power in professional relationships**
- **To examine and understand issues of sexuality and attraction between nurses and patients**

Introduction

Nurses cannot help being involved with people at all sorts of levels. People, when they are ill, are not simply people who have a particular disease or illness. They are also experiencing all sorts of psychological and perhaps even spiritual problems. Even though it is sometimes easy to consider illness and health as simply changes in bodily functions, a few moments reflection proves this not to be the case. We do not need to develop a complicated theoretical debate in order to drive this point home. Anyone who has been ill in any way will know it to be self-evident. To suffer is to experience some sort of change in self-concept and a change in the way we relate to others.

Nurses, then, do not simply look after people's bodies. They look after the whole person. Perhaps even the term 'looking after' is a dated one. Recently, nurses have come to appreciate that they do not act as surrogate parents to adults who have adopted a child role. Becoming ill or in any way dysfunctional does not mean that people automatically regress or become more childlike. More often, it is the case that the medical system that 'cares' for them forces them into such a role. Consider how you feel while sitting waiting to see your GP, for example. Do you see the meeting as one of equals? Are you nervous – not just of what the GP might say – but about the business of sitting and talking to her or him? In the past, it was probably true that all health professionals exercised a considerable amount of power over other people. Gradually, that power balance is changing in favour of the client or patient.

Nurses, then, in considering *how* to work with counselling skills should first consider their relationship towards clients and patients. The relationship should, as far as possible, be an *empowering* one rather than one in which the nurse 'takes over' the client or patient.

We turn, now, to situations in which nurses might use counselling skills.

ACTIVITY BOX 3.1

- Write down as many situations that you can think of in which the use of counselling skills in nursing might be appropriate.

The process of talking and listening in a sympathetic and empowering way can be used in a wide range of situations in nursing. A short list might include the following:

- during health care checks in health centres and GP practices
- whilst talking to people in accident and emergency departments
- while admitting people to hospital

- prior to operations and other surgical interventions
- when people are particularly upset or anxious
- while talking with relatives
- in helping colleagues to come to terms with loss or change.

Perhaps, in the end, counselling skills can be used in *most* situations and, in a later chapter, we will explore this possibility.

The idea of using a 'set of skills' at all, in the sense, raises problems. If we think of most everyday conversations, we will notice that what marks them out is their spontaneity. We do not normally stop to think of exactly the right words to use, any more than we usually stop to consider whether or not we are listening properly. In using counselling skills, we have to stop and *reflect* on what we do. At first glance, this may appear to be a highly artificial thing to do. On the other hand, most of the skills that we use in everyday life are awkward to use to begin with. As we continue to use them, we use them in a more fluid and easy fashion. Counselling skills are not dissimilar. At first, we are likely to feel awkward and even embarrassed about using them. Concentrating too hard on how we talk and listen to others can even lead us to stopping altogether – the very act of noticing how we talk and listen makes us too self-conscious to continue. After a while, though, this stage passes and we learn to incorporate into our everyday repertoire of behaviour those skills that suit both us and the people with whom we work. To this end, there are no 'formulas' for good and effective counselling. There are no particular words or phrases that must be learned. The nub of the process is learning how to listen and how to focus your attention and effort on the other person's situation.

DIALOGUE 3.1

This conversation takes place between a nurse and a 16-year-old boy who is about to have an appendectomy.

'Do you know much about my operation?'
'Yes, I've looked after people who've had the same sort of operation.'
'I'm worried about it, that's all.'
'What, in particular, are you worried about?'
'Not coming round from the anaesthetic!'
'You're worried about that . . .'
'Sort of. I know lots of people who've had the same sort of operation and they were all right.'

'So you agree that you should be, too?'
'Yes. I guess so. (Laughs) It's stupid, really, but I get nervous, that's all.'
'I appreciate that. Is there anything else you're worried about.'
'Nothing much. Only something silly.'
'What's that?'
'Nah. It's OK.'
'Well, I don't want to push you but feel free to talk about anything.'
'Well. It's just the scar. Will it be very big?'
'No. About an inch or so.'
'Oh! That's OK. I thought it would be a great big sort of gash down my side! I was worried that people at school would laugh at me.'
'You feel a bit better about it now?'
'Yes. Thanks a lot! You're not too bad here, you know!'
'Thank *you*!'

QUESTIONS ABOUT THE DIALOGUE

- What skills do *you* think were being demonstrated by the nurse?
- What did the nurse do that allowed the boy to talk?
- What would you have done differently?

REFLECTIONS

The question arises as to whether or not patients coming into hospital are tacitly giving their permission to be counselled. Many patient's needs assessment forms ask that patients be encouraged to reveal quite a lot about themselves. Is it right to ask people, for example, who are being admitted for surgery for a duodenal ulcer, about their spiritual or even sexual life? Do patients being asked fairly personal questions really exercise choice in whether or not to answer these sorts of questions? One point of view would be, given the circumstances of being in hospital and being cared for by professionals who occupy a dominant position in relation to the patient, that the patient has little real ability to say 'no' to certain sorts of enquiries. However much people are reassured that failure to take part in an assessment procedure will not affect the quality of the care they receive, it seems likely that many will feel somewhat pressurised. For some, too, the process of being a patient means 'giving in' or 'giving themselves up' to the medical and nursing professions.

Why should patients find hospitals so daunting? What is it about the working culture of health professionals that creates such a frequently inhibitive environment for patients? What ideas and principles have influenced and allowed such cultures to develop?

To discover the answers to such questions we must look at the historical factors and themes that have influenced the cultural development of health care over the past 300 years.

Fundamental principles and ideas

Although much of care delivery is now based on a holistic view of the patient, research suggests that the remnants of a more 'rigid' and inflexible approach can still be found (Mackay 1989, 1993, Kitson 1991). We will begin by considering the thinking of René Descartes, a seventeenth-century philosopher whose ideas have greatly influenced the method and organisation of Western health care.

SEPARATING MIND FROM BODY

During the seventeenth century, a revolution of ideas took place that challenged the accepted methods of thinking, it was known as the Renaissance. It was a period of great intellectual growth; the boundaries of knowledge were constantly challenged as innovative thinking and enquiry caused academics to question traditional propositions. Descartes was a central figure in many philosophical and mathematical debates but devoted much of his attention to investigating the relationship between the mind and the body. What emerged from this was a radical enquiry which confronted and challenged all convention and thinking about the relationship between the mind and body.

Prior to the Renaissance, the dominant way of thinking was that all actions were controlled and ordained by divine will. Descartes contested these themes, believing that the mind could best be seen as autonomous and free from external influence. Such reasoning was based on the notion that the body was directly comparable to a machine because both had parts which could break and need repair. The final stage in Descartes' argument continued this stand and maintained that the body was most accessibly studied by reducing it into components

and sections. Initially, this took the form of splitting the body into systems but, with scientific advancement, has progressed to the point that we can now study at the submolecular level.

Descartes' philosophical view of the split between the mind and the body is known as 'Cartesian dualism'. By attempting to give philosophical rigour and analysis to a conceptual split between mind and body, Descartes greatly influenced the method of scientific medical enquiry; it provided the impetus for ever increasing specialisation and treating parts of the body rather than the body as a whole.

Cartesian dualism placed the body firmly in the medical domain and gave licence to a reductionistic approach (that is, studying the body by theoretically 'reducing' it into ever smaller parts), which rapidly gained popularity as the most scientifically acceptable method of discovering new knowledge. This mode of practice has contributed greatly to the way in which medical research has developed and is carried out. Humankind has benefited from this and the effectiveness of modern medical therapies and treatments certainly has its roots in the ideas that Descartes offered.

Medical specialists offer a breadth of knowledge and expertise that could never be found in the generic practitioner. In terms of an example, oncology would never have existed if the pathology of cancer had not been reduced to the intricate physiology of the cell. Emerging from this is a strong argument in support of the essential themes that underpin Cartesian thinking; if medicine's main aim is to confront the disease process and do everything realistically possible to achieve a cure, then Descartes' ideas provide a valid basis for such an endeavour.

However, while such an approach (often referred to as the 'medical model') may be accepted as the mode of operation for doctors, it is open to scrutiny whether such an approach is suitable to nursing.

THE MEDICAL MODEL AND NURSING PRACTICE

It has already been said that the chief purpose of the medical model is to address the disease process; the means of achieving this meet with a successful end if the patient is cured. However, when these themes become the basis for nursing practice, it creates a working culture that can lead to the patient being seen as a condition rather than a person. This shift from the patient as a valued subject to a devalued object is found in many of the ward-based activities operated when nursing care is influenced by the medical model. Pearson and Vaughan (1986: 25) provide an erudite and reflective comment upon the relationship between the medical model and nursing:

> However, the biomedical model is reductionistic and dualistic in approach – it both reduces the human body to a set of related parts and it separates the mind from the body – and its common use in nursing is no longer appropriate. It is not geared to the needs of individuals and its dominant effect on health care has led to it being used in the interest of health professionals rather than those who seek, need or are directed to health care. Therefore, it can no longer be acknowledged as a possible choice when nursing teams are selecting a model for practice.

Even today, when nursing models and individualised care are playing an increasingly prominent role, it is still common to find work organised according to tasks, routine and physical care giving. This approach finds particular prominence in the organisation of work in wards for care of the elderly. Kitson (1991: 23) comments upon this lack of distinction between the medical and nursing frameworks by stating:

> When one considers the corresponding nursing care model, which could have served as the theoretical framework for the geriatric nursing care model, a major problem arises, namely that nursing does not have an operational model independent of the medical model.

This failure to develop a framework which establishes those characteristics of nursing that are separate and distinct from medicine cannot be blamed solely on the dominant nature of the medical model. To use terms such as 'autonomous', 'responsible' and 'accountable' in relation to nursing practice seems quite facile when the medical model can hold such influence over the approach used for the delivery of care. Nurses must accept a degree of culpability for the level of inertia which has allowed this position to continue and prosper. Again, Kitson (1991: 220) comments upon this professional indictment by stating:

> Nursing practice seemed content to follow in the wake of medical innovation and change.

In consequence, nursing was unable to consider seriously the complexities involved in providing care. Nursing also failed to determine its essential components and failed to build a framework that would ensure the goal of care was achieved in the practice setting.

It seems hardly credible that nursing could have allowed itself to have been so affected by the themes underpinning medicine. Even today's so-called professional advances seem to support the ethos of the medical model; as Kendrick (1997: 3) states,

> Yet increasingly, advancing practice does not seem concerned with the skills I have visited here. Today, advanced practice seems to be focused on increasing nurses' technical expertise. This usually involves nurses adopting 'tasks' that had previously been performed exclusively by doctors. It seems strange that, after spending so long moving from care based on 'task allocation', that we now embrace 'tasks' doctors no longer want and say it advances nursing practice.

The issues we have discussed here find particular focus when considered in terms of the influence they have had upon interprofessional relationships between doctors and nurses; this, in turn, has a cumulative effect upon the way in which patients are view and cared for.

DOCTOR, NURSE, PATIENT

The nurse–doctor relationship lies at the very heart of health care delivery. Traditionally, this association has involved the nurse giving care based upon the doctor's orders. Such thinking is graphically supported by the following quotation from Chadwick and Tadd (1992: 49):

> Characteristically, the doctor has been portrayed as 'all knowing' and powerful; the nurse as careful, unselfish, obedient and submissive; and the patient as helpless and utterly trusting.

Although nurses and doctors are key conduits in health care delivery, research indicates that the lay public and, indeed, doctors themselves, continue to see a vast difference in the status and power that each group enjoys (Holloway 1992). This has helped to maintain an image that portrays nurses as passive and acquiescent while doctors are assertive and dominant (Kendrick 1995b).

ACTIVITY BOX 3.2

■ List reasons to explain why doctors have more status and power than nurses.

There are many possible reasons to explain the level of disparity which exists between doctors and nurses. Seeking to find a key theme to explain the different power base that each professional group holds, Turner (1986) argues that nursing's traditional allegiance to servility has allowed doctors to prescribe and delegate the activities of care giving. Part of the reason for the continued existence of this power-based scenario is that nursing is still seen as something which is essentially 'feminine' and concerned with caring and nurturing. Conversely, medicine is associated with masculine themes of curing, science, objectivity and assertiveness. To understand the reasons for these different influences and why nursing is seen as subservient to medicine, we must take a brief look at some theoretical and historical developments.

GOOD NURSE – GOOD WOMAN

Florence Nightingale vehemently believed that nursing was a female endeavour and she equated the idea of being a good nurse with that of being a 'good' woman. This placed a great deal of emphasis upon those virtues which were seen as genteel and feminine; principal among these were sobriety and chastity. Equipped with such moral steadfastness, Nightingale thought that nursing could best serve and preserve the overriding maxim that a nurse's first duty was to do the patient no harm. Such thinking is well-meaning but lacks rigour and focus when viewed in the light of professional practice with patients. Much of health care causes an initial harm that is justified by a net effect which should produce good. An illustration often used to describe this theme is an intramuscular injection; whilst the syringe entering tissue causes pain, this is usually outweighed by the therapeutic worth of the drug which is introduced. Taking this to its logical conclusion, nurses cannot say that their interventions will never cause the patient harm; it is more accurate to say that the risk of harm should be kept to a minimum and always be justified by the probability of increased benefit.

Garmarnikow (1978: 116) examined Nightingale's writing and clearly illustrates the emphasis which is placed upon female virtues as a basis for the moral aptitude required for nursing:

> Nightingale insisted on the existence of a close link between nursing and femininity, the latter being defined by a specific combination of moral qualities which differentiated men from women. The success of nursing reforms depended primarily, according to Nightingale, on cultivating the 'feminine' character, rather than on training and education.

The so-called 'feminine' traits to which Nightingale appeals are those that have traditionally reinforced much of the negative imagery which has dwarfed and fettered women's position in relation to men. This is mirrored by the traditional association which places women as caring and nurturing figures who preserve the homestead and bring up children. Such themes have been developed by some commentators and applied to the therapeutic aspects of nurse–patient interaction. In a seminal paper, Lewin (1977: 91) draws parallels between the role of the women in the domicile and that of the nurse caring for patients:

> The identification of nursing with femaleness derives not only from its 'unselfish service' component, but also from the importance of physical nurturance, and a sort of material intimacy, which also enter into the image of nursing work. The close acquaintance of the nurse with the messy details of illness is not unlike the mother's necessary involvement with infantile bodily functions.

The central thrust of Lewin's argument is that certain nursing acts resemble the way in which a mother cares for an infant or newborn. This is mirrored in nursing when practitioners have to deal with aesthetically undesirable features, such as faeces, urine or vomit. Such themes are further supported by Lawler (1991: 223) who states:

> One of the salient features of nurses' work that closely links it to women's traditional roles is the similarity between body care and mothering.

Commenting upon the analogy between nursing and motherhood, Kendrick (1995a: 240) states:

> Both situations demand responsible actions but the key feature is the emphasis which is

placed upon maternity, femaleness and being a woman. Such themes are seen as exclusively female because of the male world view which dominates society; this is mirrored by the disempowered standing which women have traditionally suffered in scenarios with men – within either the domestic or clinical environment.

Taking the argument a stage further, we have already said that nursing's concern with the themes associated with caring is subservient to the scientific, cure-orientated features of medicine. Commenting upon the influence that this distinction brings to interprofessional relations between doctors and nurses, Adshead and Dickenson (1993: 167) state:

> If nursing is defined as being about caring and medicine about curing, medicine will continue to be seen as more important. If the role of the female paradigm profession of nursing is seen as caring, the old stereotype of the nurse as doctor's 'helpmeet' will be revived. Caring is likely to be seen as less important than curing because we fear death and wrongly attribute to medicine the power to cure us of mortality.

ACTIVITY BOX 3.3

In the light of what you have read, consider the following scenario based upon a real example from practice. All names used are fictitious and certain features have been changed to preserve the anonymity of those involved.

A series of investigations have shown Bill to have a particularly aggressive form of bowel cancer with secondary deposits in the liver, bone, and some spread to the brain. The consultant surgeon, Simon Smith, has performed a colostomy to try and alleviate some of Bill's discomfort; however, the overall prognosis is dire.

At the end of a ward round, the team are discussing Bill's position and Janice, a staff nurse, comments, 'Bill was telling me today that nobody has discussed the findings of the latest scan with him. Then he asked if it would be all right to book a holiday in Portugal for next spring – I just know he is near to asking whether or not he will get over this.'

Simon Smith interjects 'Well, if he does ask about his prognosis, refer him to me and I'll break the news as gently as I can.'

Janice looks unsettled and challenges Simon's position – 'Look Simon, if Bill asks me a direct question about his death I feel a bit awkward about shirking responsibility and passing it on to you'.

Simon gives Janice a firm and direct answer- 'you are not shirking your responsibility. This man has extensive cancer and I've done everything clinically possible to address it – this has been unsuccessful. Therefore, as his doctor, I have the clinical mandate to tell him that the only feasible path left is to try and control his symptoms and make life physically bearable during the time he has left.'

- Write down what this example tells you about the power relationship between doctors and nurses.
- State whether or not you have experienced similar situations in your own practice.
- If you have had an experience like this, write down how you dealt with it and how the incident left you feeling.

REFLECTIONS

There will be some nurses who read this case study and argue vehemently that they would never let a doctor stop them telling a patient about 'bad news' (Kendrick 1995b). Conversely, there will be nurses who closely identify with the case study and Janice's dilemma with the attitude of Simon Smith, the consultant surgeon. Other commentators have made similar claims when writing about relationships between doctors and nurses; for example, after discussing various scenarios of real conflicts from practice, Brown *et al.* (1992: 71) state:

> Readers who do find these incidents extraordinary will not share this chapter's working assumption that there are at present serious inequalities in the relationship between doctors and nurses.

Such scenarios certainly curtail opportunites to counsel Bill and explore the future honestly. This sort of development can negatively influence care delivery and contribute, reinforce and underpin the themes listed below; this can, cumulatively, make patients feel dwarfed, childlike and disempowered:

- frequent invasion of personal space
- unfamiliar routines
- reduced ability to achieve activities of daily living
- hidden rules
- fear of medical procedures
- lack of privacy.

What we have discovered here are the historical and cultural dimensions and developments that have helped to forge, and still influence, the delivery of modern health care. Even before nurses think about offering counselling to patients, it is useful to understand the powerful influence of culture upon professional dynamics. Some patients will feel comfortable with care delivery that mirrors the approach of the medical model. For them, the most important thing is to get the physical problem addressed and get out of hospital. Patients who prefer this sort of approach usually feel less comfortable with the idea of baring their soul in the interests of holistic care – that is their choice and their privilege. Other people feel daunted by coming into hospital and need the opportunity to talk about themselves and express their wants, fears and needs.

The key issue is choice, giving patients the freedom to decide how their care should be framed and delivered in the essence of holism, and this should be the focus of our professional endeavour.

INTERPERSONAL ISSUES

What should a counsellor do if he or she is attracted to a client? What should he or she do if the client becomes attracted to the counsellor? These questions are vitally important and deserve focused consideration. We will begin by exploring the difficult issues that arise when a counsellor is attracted to a client or vice versa.

NB The term 'counsellor–client relationship' is used inclusively here and applies equally to the nurse–patient relationship where the nurse is using counselling skills

NATURAL ATTRACTION

A primal human feature is the facility to find other individuals attractive. On one level, this has importance as a biological theme. Taking this further, attraction is an important starting point in human sexuality; without it, the propagation of the human species would never have been possible. Of course, this is reducing sexuality to its most essential *raison d'être*.

Human sexuality is a complex phenomenon that goes way beyond the boundaries of procreation. It rises above the heterosexual conclave of marriage – what Luther compared to a hospital that cures lust (Zeldin 1994) – and figures buoyantly as a key characteristic in the human condition.

Sexuality and attraction is not confined to the young, nubile and fertile; it is something that exists and can thrive across the lifespan. This is given sharp focus by Stuart-Hamilton (1994: 125), who states:

> It is a commonplace observation that the media portray sex as being for the young and slim, and ageist humour dictates that older people wanting a sex life are either 'dirty old men' or ugly and desperate. Even those older people whom the media have labelled as 'sexy' are chosen because they do not 'look their age'. Accordingly, the elderly do not receive support from everyday sources that wanting a sex life is normal and healthy.

Thus, human beings have the facility to find others attractive throughout life, and this is not restricted to any given category of age. This, however, does not mean an automatic link between attraction and sexual activity; this point is at the centre of our discussion. It is natural that, on occasion, a counsellor and a client will form a therapeutic relationship that is charged with sexual energy. This is the essence of being human, every now and then we may meet someone who sends our emotions into a swirling quagmire. The central point is what we do with those emotions and what should be the focus for such powerful energy; these issues cast down a gauntlet to the counsellor.

HUMAN VULNERABILITY

A key point in the counsellor–client relationship is that the client is vulnerable and does not enter the relationship in the same way that dynamics are forged in everyday social milieus; for example, the relationship between counsellor and counselled is hardly the same as how people meet in, for example, a pub, club, restaurant or other popular meeting place; nor are the terms of engagement the same in the counsellor–client relationship as in ordinary social interaction. This, by definition, creates an arena whereby the counsellor is placed in a position of power; understanding the basis of this power is important for helping to understand the dynamics that frame such interaction, especially when this involves nurses exercising counselling skills.

BEYOND POWER

Nurses use counselling skills in many different settings. Patients are, by definition, sick and often vulnerable. The very process of entering hospital or being cared for may conjure different images for different people. Some patients see hospital as a place of safety where illness or trauma will be addressed, others see it as a reflection of their own mortality and hear the ringing of the death knoll.

Added to this, hospitals have their own hidden agendas and rituals that can make patients feel disempowered and as though they should passively acquiesce to set norms and rules (Walsh and Ford 1989). There are many examples that illustrate this; however, among the most bizzare is that we expect patients to wear their night attire during the day.

Just place yourself in the patient's position; you are really worried about something and want to talk it through with someone. You sit at the side of a bed at 10 o'clock in the morning, wearing your night clothes, and the choice of people you have to talk to are busily running round wearing crisp, starched uniforms. How would you feel? Uniforms, by their nature, convey an image of authority, while pyjamas, nighties and dressing gowns all suggest passivity. After all, night attire would be the last sort of clothing you would choose to wear to be assertive.

All of these issues help to create an environment that places the nurse–patient relationship in a context of power. The type of power a nurse has is traditonally referred to as 'expert social power' (French and Raven 1959). A key feature of this sort of power is that patients are thought to trust nurses because it is their professional aim to uphold and, as far as possible, advocate for the 'best interests' of patients; also, nurses hold expert social power because patients perceive them as correct (Penner 1978). This is quite different to the sort of power that exists between a customer and a salesperson because sales are often linked to very healthy commissions – nurses do not work for these sort of incentives. Classical research also suggests that this lack of financial entanglement adds to nurses' truthworthiness (Janis *et al.* 1959).

To recap, patients may be vulnerable for a host of reasons:

- Patients are, by definition, ill, and this can bring with it associated worries that add to the individual's vulnerability.
- Being in hospital may bring with it a fear and realisation of patients' own mortality.
- Hospitals have a specific culture that can make some patients feel isolated; there are certainly specific routines and traditions that frame the day and patients are expected to conform to these.
- Patients perceive nurses to be authoritative figures who will represent their best interests.

What emerges from this is that being a patient can be a frightening experience. When patients are placed in this sort of scenario it can make great demands on their emotional equilibrium. Moreover, the process of counselling a patient can be an intense and deeply powerful experience that can create and unleash a potent cocktail where those involved feel attracted to each other. The key point is, as we keep reinforcing, the patient's vulnerability.

INTIMACY AND VULNERABILITY

The nurse does not meet the patient as an emotional equal but, instead, at a time when the patient is experiencing a life event. A central purpose of the relationship is to help patients transcend that event, or, if that is not possible, to create an arena where they may be supported in facing the inevitability of death. Feeling attracted to patients is sometimes part of the baggage that nurses carry for caring for people during such a period of crisis. It is impossible to create an empathic relationship based on authenticity that does not engage the emotions.

The nurse–patient relationship is also unique because it often means care delivery that involves a physical intimacy; Stewart (1983: 10) comments upon this aspect in the following way:

> Procedures involving the sexual areas of the body present even greater difficulties. Contact (and this is not necessarily physical; exposure to the eyes is a very potent from of contact) in these areas is generally reserved for a specific purpose and for specific people. Nurses, when they have overcome their shyness, can become rather blasé about intimate contact (including exposure of the patient) without fully realising the emotional impact this may have on the patient.

Lawler (1991: 113) gives further focus to these themes:

> As part of their work, nurses must negotiate not only normal social boundaries when they touch others (patients), but, because the body is heavily inscribed with meaning – much of it sexual – nurses' work is socially fragile, and they must learn ways to make their work manageable.

Taking these themes further, a position may arise where nurses are involved in delivering a care package that can, at one moment, involve touching a patient's most intimate bodily parts, while later offering counselling skills that impact upon the patient's emotional milieu. Such scenarios, research reveals, can certainly fuel the flame that helps patients feel attracted to nurses (Assay and Herbert 1983). Moreover, wearing the mantle of professionalism does not make a nurse immune to the power of interpersonal attractiveness – to argue otherwise is to deny an essential element of human sexuality.

We are concentrating here on the patients' vulnerability but 'being vulnerable' is something that affects every human being at various times in life. When a nurse is emotionally vulnerable, it makes it all the more difficult to 'walk away' from an emotional encounter with a patient whom he or she may find attractive. When we feel vulnerable there is often a need to feel valued, respected and needed; patients frequently offer this. When such themes are coupled with a physical attraction, then interpersonal dynamics become very difficult to focus and handle.

A major problem is that the profession of nursing has been very slow to explore the issue of interpersonal attractiveness between nurses and patients. If such themes could be addressed in an open manner, it might lead to discussion and debate about something that is a vital feature of human encounters. We all know of patients who have asked nurses out; equally, we all know nurses who have accepted. Moreover, who among us can honestly claim, hand on heart, that they have never found a patient attractive – and how did we handle those emotions once they arose? This is a debate that clearly needs a much wider airing.

However, the essential point is that the patient is the focus of care giving and that care has to be delivered in an accountable and responsible manner. It is difficult to envisage accountability sitting comfortably with a relationship that crosses profes-sional borders, where sexual energy can become the dominant force.

To support such notions, we have already seen, in the previous chapter, that counselling sometimes involves helping the patient to make decisions that may cause certain emotional discomfort. If a nurse is emotionally involved with a patient, it may be difficult to create an arena where such things can be broached. In essence, emotional, sensual involvement with patients can compromise professional judgement; this cannot be reconcilable with the essential elements of cogent counselling.

This is not based on a dogmatic view of morality – we freely acknowledge that nurses sometimes find patients attractive and vice versa; however, when such themes develop in an arena where patients have a right to, and nurses a duty to provide, the best possible care, relationships charged by frissons of the erotic may compromise such aims (we shall return to this subject again in Chapter 9).

ACTIVITY BOX 3.4

Reflect for a few moments on conversations that you have had with patients in different situations. Think, then, about the sorts of situations which you would not handle very well. Think, then, about the sorts of situations that you think you would handle well. What are the main differences between the two? To help you with this activity, here are some situations to think about:

- An elderly woman wants to talk to you about the fact that she is dying.
- A teenage girl needs to talk to you about the fact that she has missed a period.
- A 9-year-old boy asks you what the operation on his umbilical hernia involves.

Conclusion

This chapter has considered aspects of counselling that occur in nursing situations. We need to think about whether or not nursing and counselling are so closely linked together as to make them inseparable or whether or not counselling is a separate sort of activity. If we decide that counselling and nursing are part of the same activity, then we need to think even more carefully about *training* issues. How are nurses trained to be counsellors? If, on the other hand, we decide that nursing and counselling are two separate activities, then we may want to consider *which* nurses should do counselling. If only certain types of nurses are to work as counsel-lors, how are we to decide which ones, who makes that decision and how are such nurses to be selected and then trained? Given the cultural dimensions of practice, power, and interprofessional and inter-personal relationships, such questions certainly demand considered answers.

4 PLANNING COUNSELLING

CHAPTER AIMS

- To consider the structure of the counselling relationship
- To identify some of the environmental considerations

Introduction

It is useful to consider two sorts of counselling: *informal* and *formal*. These distinctions are meant to convey the two ways in which nurses might use counselling skills in their everyday work. The informal type of counselling is that which every nurse does every time she talks to a patient in hospital or in the community with a view to *helping* them. This sort of informal counselling includes, at least, the following sorts of situations:

- explaining what an operation is going to be for
- discussing changes in medication
- reassuring the person who is upset
- talking to patients' relatives

and so on.

More formal counselling takes place when the nurse decides to meet with a patient (or with a colleague) for the express purpose of talking about the other person's problems. Formal counselling might involve a nurse who has a formal counselling qualification or it might be undertaken by a nurse who has had considerable experience of talking about problems.

The idea of *structure* in the counselling relationship is useful. Almost all nurses are busy and have to decide how to use their time. Structure can help to use time most effectively. There are other advantages to structure. First, structure can help the client to be aware of how long any given counselling discussion will take place. It can also indicate to him or her how *many* counselling discussions there will be. Second, it helps to make sure that the counselling

discussion does not simply become 'chatting'. The point of counselling is to remain reasonably focused and to make sure that the time is used to help the client. Third, structure can help both parties to make sense of what is happening. Most people, in most aspects of life, benefit from structure of this sort.

Definitions

A simple structure for a series of counselling conversations might be as follows:

- the exploratory phase
- the goal-setting phase
- the identification of means of goal achievement
- work on achieving goals
- evaluating the work/setting new goals.

THE EXPLORATORY PHASE

In this phase, the client is encouraged to talk very generally about anything that he or she wants to. This is the 'storytelling' phase. That is not to say that the client is making things up but rather to convey the idea that he or she is telling the counsellor about his or her world, about how he or she sees things and how he or she identifies problem areas. Although many problems are common to many of us – financial problems, relationship problems, self-identity problems, to name but three sorts – we all *conceive* of these in different sorts of ways. It is probably a mistake to assume that what is a problem for one person is necessarily a problem for another. Likewise, it is a mistake to assume that something that appears minor to the counsellor is minor for the client. Two examples will suffice here. A person being counselled by one of the authors (P.B.), many years ago, revealed that he was a rubber fetishist: he found sexual pleasure in dressing up in rubber clothes. The author felt that this was likely to be the 'core' of his problems and continued to pursue the issue with the client. This was because the counsellor felt that being a rubber fetishist would be a problem for *him*, the counsellor, if he enjoyed this type of activity. In practice, however, the client's 'real' problems were to do with finances; he did not find being a rubber fetishist a problem at all! The second example is of a client whose budgie had died. In this case, the fact was fairly quickly glossed over and the counsellor was keen to move on to other 'more important' topics. In the end, though, it became apparent that the client's 'real' problem was the issue of bereavement for the budgie. It is something of a prime rule in counselling and psychotherapy that the counsellor does not assume that the client's problems are the counsellor's and that the counsellor does not assume that his or her *own* problems are shared by the client.

THE GOAL-SETTING PHASE

Out of the first, exploratory, phase comes the first glimpses of issues that the client worries about. The client may identify, fairly quickly, what the main problems are. Alternatively, they may be revealed very slowly, sometimes in the guise of something else. A client may, for example, talk of not being able to get along with their parents and/or his or her workmates. Later, though, it transpires that what the client 'really' worries about is getting along with himself or herself.

It is helpful if the various problems are addressed, at some point, in terms of *goals* to be achieved. This is not always discussed in the literature. Some authorities feel that counselling should be an open-ended 'process' affair. However, nurses' time is limited and it makes good sense to consider goal setting as a way of structuring the counselling relationship. Goals can be long and short term. The long-term ones are likely to be less specific than the short-term ones. However, all goals should be clearly stated in behavioural terms. A goal should be achievable, identify a single state or behaviour and be approved of by the client. It should also be realistic. It is one thing to *want* to undertake certain

life changes, it is quite another to achieve them. One of the counsellor's roles is to help the client to set realistic and achievable goals.

French (1993), discussing the work of Gerard Egan, offers a range of useful strategies for helping clients to think about the goals they want to achieve, as follows:

- Ask future-oriented questions, or try to frame questions in ways that ask about how things could be, how things would be better and how things could be different to the way they are now.
- Help clients find models, which means help clients to identify people who they respect and explore how these people would deal with the issues.
- Review better times, by looking at instances in the past where issues were resolved satisfactorily or conditions were more favourable.
- Help clients to get involved in new experiences, and discover different outlooks on life. Changes in leisure activities, occupation, lifestyle, routines, location, friends or partners may bring fresh perspectives and even a new appreciation of these aspects of the present scenario.
- Use writing approaches. This is a method of clarifying thoughts and communication with oneself in an almost objective way. The creative element of writing poetry, short stories and letters can enable the development of imagination concerning a particular scenario.
- Use fantasy. This is a powerful way of achieving and developing imagination. Some people find it easier to fantasise than others, and one of the inhibitions to fantasising is that it is not bound by reality and can seem to be ridiculous at times. When developing this skill, it is important for the counsellor to be accepting and tolerant of another person's outlandish ideas.

THE IDENTIFICATION OF MEANS OF GOAL ACHIEVEMENT

After the goals have been set, it is necessary to identify the means by which they can be achieved. This can be done in various ways. First, it can be done simply by talking about what has to happen next. Second, it can be done through the process known as 'brainstorming'. Here the client and counsellor sit down and imagine all the possible and impossible ways in which goals may be achieved. This is a 'free form' sort of activity that need not be bounded by time and which may take more than one session to achieve. Once all the possible and unlikely means have been identified, the client and counsellor identify the ones that *will* be used. This, again, is often a question of bringing some compromise to bear. It may also be a phase in which the goals are reassessed slightly and modified. Again, it is important to be skilled in the 'art of the possible' and to aim both at goals and at means of goal achievement that can be achieved.

WORK ON ACHIEVING GOALS

The next stage, for the counsellor, is a supportive one. During the next few weeks and months (and even years) the client works on achieving goals via the identified means. During this time, the counsellor simply 'stays with' the client and encourages and supports him. Again, during this phase, it may be necessary to modify some of the goals that have been set. It is important, though, not to modify goals *too quickly*. Sometimes, it is easier to modify goals than to work at achieving them. Here, again, the counsellor's role is to help to keep the client on track.

EVALUATING THE WORK/SETTING NEW GOALS

The final stage in the structure is that of evaluating the work that has been done to achieve the goals. Sometimes, this will mean that the client takes encouragement that goals have been achieved. Sometimes, it is simply a breathing space in which both the client and the counsellor look back over what has been achieved towards the goals. Once some of the goals *have* been achieved, it seems likely that some new goals will need to be set. This may become a continuous process, depending on the relationship and time frame that exists between the client and the counsellor. It is important to acknowledge that all counselling relationships have to end. Counselling is not best thought of as a totally open-ended process that has no limit. Indeed, it is often better to set a time limit on the relationship at the *start* of the relationship.

DIALOGUE 4.1

The exploratory phase

'So, what's happening in your life at the moment?'
'Well, I'm getting on better with my parents. I'm

working – at least for the moment. And this hospital stay is likely to change all that, unfortunately.'
'When you say "change *all* that", what do you mean?'
'I'll start falling out with my parents again. We always fall out when I'm not working. Basically, we all get on each other's nerves. And they think that I didn't work hard enough at school and college.'
'What do you think?'
'I think I did what I could. Sort of. I suppose I didn't do enough, really....'

The goal-setting phase

'So, out of all this, what do you want to do?'
'Lots of things ...'
'What are the most important things?'
'Working, studying again, getting on with my parents ...'
'OK, let's start with working and studying ...'

The identification of means of goal achievement

'So, how are you going to do some of this?'
'What do you mean?'
'What has got to happen to help you get a job? And then, what has got to happen to get you back studying again?' Let's deal with the job question first ...'

Work on achieving goals

'What has been happening since we last met?
'I've been to four interviews and I've got two more.'
'That's good. What are your feelings about the two new interviews?'
'Not bad. I've got a good chance with one, I think. Not so good with the other but it's not a job that I'm all that keen on.'
'What preparation have you made for the 'good' one, then?'
'I've got a new suit! That's a start! I've been reading a lot, too. I've also got a book about being interviewed. That should help.'
'It certainly should. That all sounds excellent.'

Evaluating the work/setting new goals

'Where have we got to, now?'
'I've got the job and I start at college next October. The college isn't quite what I had in mind.'
'But it means you're studying again?'
'It does. I suppose it's not a bad idea.'

'It's what we've talked about a lot. It sounds good.'
'Thanks. I think it is, really!'

Questions about the dialogue

Read through the above dialogue again and consider the following questions.

- What were the 'best' interventions made by the counsellor?
- What would you change about the way the counselling was managed?
- Did the counsellor *lead* and, if so, is this acceptable?
- How would *you* have counselled this person?

REFLECTIONS

The question of *leading* in counselling is an interesting and important one. In the *client-centred* approach to counselling, advocated by Carl Rogers (1951), the aim was never to lead but always to take the lead from the client. Essential to the client-centred approach to counselling is the idea that the client always knows what is best for himself or herself and it is the counsellor's task not to offer advice or suggestions but to encourage the client to find his or her way through their problems. This approach has been very much to the fore for the last three decades. It is, however, time-consuming. It also means that the counsellor has to have a particularly optimistic view of people and their ability to self-direct. Nurses have to work to tight time-schedules and it seems to the authors that a *mixture* of leading and allowing the client to lead is a reasonable working arrangement. The above dialogue illustrates the way in which the client, for the most part, decides on the path that he takes through the things that he wants to do. On the other hand, the counsellor is prepared to 'nudge' him a little and this seems to help him to get back on track and to remain in touch with what he is doing. The question here is 'to what degree is it *right* to "nudge" a person in this way?' If you believe, totally, that people are always self-directing, then you are unlikely to approve of nudging. If, on the other hand, you believe that, to some degree, people are determined by the society in which they live and affected by the people with whom they come into contact, you might more readily accept the idea that most people need a little direction in their lives and that such direction might come from a counsellor.

Freedom to decide

The vexed issue of whether a counsellor should 'nudge' a person or whether that person should be given freedom to 'lead self' is closely linked to the concept of autonomy. We have already explored the notion of autonomy (Chapter 1); it is impossible to be 'self-governing' in the purest sense of the word since each person is influenced by so many other considerations. How many times have you really wanted to escape from the pressures of everyday life only to be limited by the demands of family or work? The simple truth is that we cannot be free to self-govern because of the barriers life and circumstances place before us.

Patients in hospital, for reasons we have already explored, often feel vulnerable. It is difficult enough dealing with everyday trials and tribulations; being cast into a strange, clinical environment hardly promotes the sort of ambience where someone would feel at ease to make important decisions about care. When nurses use counselling skills with patients, they need to consider the limitations that sickness and hospitalisation place upon patients. Something that would have caused a person no problem at all prior to illness can present major problems during periods of vulnerability.

We are not saying here that all patients passively acquiesce to the dominant norms and values of the clinical environment. On occasion, nurses do meet patients who are very assertive and wish to have total command of their care programme. However, patients can only define their best interests in so far as this fits in with what health professionals are at liberty to offer; for example, at the time of writing, it is illegal to agree to a patient's request for euthanasia. One of the authors (K.K.) often works in palliative care environments where patients occasionally make the most heart-rending pleas for help to die. When talking with these patients, it often becomes apparent that such pleas really do reflect their wishes – yet agreeing to such requests goes way beyond the limits of a nurse's professional scope. This shows that there are times when patients make requests for something that clearly cannot be delivered. At such times, it does become necessary to gently 'nudge' patients in the direction to realise that there are limits to the things that nurses can do and offer.

The questions we are considering here about whether a person should be given the absolute freedom to be self-directing or whether this should sometimes be influenced by the counsellor is closely linked with another important ethical concept – advocacy.

Acting on behalf of whom?

In recent years, advocacy has been grasped as a vital theme in health care delivery; its central purpose is to represent, safeguard and promote the interests of patients. This presents itself by practitioners becoming an 'active voice' when, for whatever reason, patients feel unable to articulate or represent their own best interests. Nursing has always embraced the notion that the patient's best interests should be paramount. This is the very essence of the professional creed and is mirrored by the following edict from the Code of Professional Conduct:

> Each registered nurse, midwife and health visitor shall act, at all times, in such a manner as to: safeguard and promote the interests of individual patients and clients. (UKCC 1992)

There is a clear link between the directive to 'promote the interests of individual patients and clients' and the intrinsic themes of advocacy. *The Concise Oxford Dictionary* (1992) defines an advocate as a 'person who pleads for another'. Such sentiments seem laudable in their abstract form. However, reconciling these elements with the reality of clinical practice is a complex and demanding task. Indeed, Brown (1985: 26) states that advocacy should be a 'means of transferring power back to the patient to enable him to control his own affairs'. Such sentiments seem laudable and reflect health care's current preoccupation with the notion of empowerment.

What we have seen, so far, is that advocacy appears to fit comfortably as a feature of the nurse's role. The notion of the nurse as the patient's advocate brings with it images of nurturing and caring that are firmly rooted in the professional ethos. Not to represent the patient's best interests seems anathema to all that is sacred to nursing traditions and values. Yet we seem to be missing a fundamental question which should be at the very heart of our enquiry, namely, 'Why should a nurse ever have to act as an advocate for the patient?' The earlier quote from Brown offers a starting point for answering this question when reference is made to 'transferring power back to the patient'. If patients are seen as equals in the delivery of health care, then why should there ever be a need to transfer 'power back'? What this reveals is that the process of delivering health care is based upon a power-laden scenario where patient vulnerability and disempowerment become the validating themes for the role of the nurse as advocate.

This is powerfully supported and echoed by Abrams (1978: 262) who states: 'The need for advocacy is the result of the failure of the health care structure to function as it should'. Thus, advocacy's shining veneer covers a lacklustre concept that is a response to the health care system's own inadequacies.

We are beginning to challenge a concept that holds centre place in much of nursing's contemporary rhetoric. If advocacy is to hold real meaning, focus and direction for nurses, then it must be viewed with a critical and enquiring gaze. Our next step will be to examine the structures which give credence and reason to the existence of advocacy in health care.

Who is best to define 'best interests'?

Despite holding an unequal position with medical colleagues, nurses have willingly grasped the role of advocate and argue that they are ideally placed to represent patients' best interests (Penn 1994). To clarify the validity of this claim, we shall briefly consider the notion of advocacy within the legal profession.

When somebody is accused of a criminal offence, he or she has a legal right to be represented by a lawyer. An onus rests upon the lawyer to represent the interests of the accused during the course of the legal process – in this way the role of advocate is fulfilled. The person accused of an alleged crime would feel that justice and due process was compromised if a lawyer was perceived as inferior or shackled by a tradition of subservience to other officers of the court. Applying these themes to a parallel scenario, how can nurses effectively fulfil the role of advocate when they hold unequal power in relation to doctors? This holds tremendous implications for the notion of 'best interests' and how they are defined.

We have already discovered that health care delivery is heavily laden with issues of power. The very need for advocacy arises from the patient entering a milieu which is both unfamiliar and disempowering.

Patients are fully aware of the power that doctors and nurses hold and are reticent about challenging the established 'norms' of patient behaviour. These themes are supported by research and are further reflected by Mackay (1993: 153), who states:

Patients are well aware of their role as the audience and as performer: they know what is expected of them. They know to be deferential when the 'great consultant' visits them and deigns to chat. They have been prepared for this great visit by the nursing staff.

This creates an environment where the patient is expected to acquiesce passively to treatment without question – the whole ambience of the clinical theme discourages notions of patient participation or active enquiry; as Penn (1994: 42) states:

> Patients are frequently reluctant to discuss their feelings with doctors and rarely challenge doctors' decisions.

What we have is a position where patients often feel vulnerable, disempowered and disenfranchised. Against this background, it is perfectly understandable that patients feel the need to have someone who can represent their best interests in a scenario which is dwarfing and threatening. The great paradox about lay persons' perceptions is that, whilst they see nurses as subservient to doctors, they still feel they can ask the nurse to represent their best interests. This phenomenon is made more poignant by patients tending to seek advocacy from the most junior of staff – often a student nurse; Thompson *et al.* (1988: 24) give this parody great resonance by drawing parallels between the process of becoming a nurse and that of becoming a patient:

> The process of becoming a nurse is in some ways similar to that of becoming a patient. The loss of a certain amount of identity, taking on a generalised role and behaving accordingly, are experiences common to nurses and patients. New nurses often feel that they are in a rigid hierarchy which relies upon rank and punitive measures rather than rationality and reason.

Given the themes we have discovered about the relation between doctors, nurses, patients and power, it seems increasingly dubious to argue that nurses can play a credible and effective role as advocates. This gains further cogency when related to terms such as 'empowerment', which are often used to describe a process that has seen the best interests of the patient realised in practice. Some commentators have taken this further and write about a utopian world where patients freely prescribe their best interests, unshackled by the constraints of vulnerability and disempowerment that we have already discussed. Reflecting this ten-dency, Murphy and Hunter (1984: 95) state:

> The professional, while obligated to act in the patient's best interests, is not permitted to define that interest in any way contrary to the patient's definition; it is not the professional but the patient that shall define what 'best interests' shall mean.

ACTIVITY BOX 4.1

If nurses, when using counselling skills, are supposed to represent the patient's 'best interests' as the patient defines them, what should our responses be in the following scenarios?

Jim is a 40-year-old alcoholic. He is being treated on a surgical ward for a pilonidal sinus. The surgery has been successful and the postoperative period uneventful. However, the surgical registrar had noticed a bottle of rum behind Jim's locker and confiscated it saying 'You can have it on discharge but you're not drinking while in my care'. Jim is distraught and pleads with a nurse saying 'Look, please get my rum back. If I start to get the 'shakes' all hell will break loose – I need that rum'.

- Would you be able to advocate for Jim in this situation?
- What response would you give to his plea?

Beryl is 55 years old and has been sectioned in an acute mental health unit. She has been suffering with depression and tried to commit suicide by taking an overdose of paracetamol. She was found by neighbours and received the antedote before any liver damage occurred. This is her 14th admission for similar problems. Each time, she receives a course of electro-convulsive therapy and is then sent into the community where she is visited monthly by a community psychiatric nurse who gives her an injection. She is constantly depressed and even after treatment she pleads to be allowed to die. One evening, she is talking to Mel, a student nurse, and says 'Why won't they let me do what I want? I just do not want to live. Why won't anybody listen to me?'

- How would you counsel Beryl if you were in Mel's position?
- Do you think it is possible to advocate for Beryl's best interests as she defines them?

REFLECTIONS

In these scenarios, it would be highly unlikely that the nurses involved would actively advocate for the patients in a way that mirrored their subjectively defined best interests. These themes are eloquently supported by Allmark and Klarzynski (1992: 34), who argue:

> An advocate should plead someone's cause as the person, and not the advocate, sees it. If a liberal lawyer pleads the cause of a neo-nazi group to have freedom of speech then this is true advocacy. A nurse is unable to provide the alcoholic with a drink, plead for the overdose not to be treated, and for the sectioned patient to be allowed to leave.

Part of the underlying trend that propagates such themes is a preoccupation among health professionals to treat patients in a way that is directly analogous to the way parents deal with a child. As we have already discovered, the combined impact of illness and being in hospital can leave patients feeling exposed and vulnerable. This situation is made worse when health professionals deal with patients in a manner that is both demeaning and patronising. When women engage in this sort of behaviour it is sometimes called matriarchy, and, in men, patriarchy. If these traits are intrinsic to the delivery of care, they can reinforce the power equation between doctors, nurses and patients. The combined influence of patriarchy and matriarchy is sometimes referred to as parentalism (Kendrick 1994). Emerging from this is an image of a 'pseudo-family', where the disempowered patient (child) conforms to the dominant wishes of the doctor (father) and nurse (mother). Such dynamics are potentially destructive and should be resisted and avoided if people are to exist in a healing and flourishing environment. This form of parentalism certainly has no role in a counselling scenario.

We have discovered here that acting as the patient's advocate may be an important part of using counselling skills as a nurse. If you believe that patients should be given *carte blanche* to define their own best interests, then acting as their advocate should be geared towards this end. However, we have explored a number of incidents where nurses did not have the freedom to fulfil patients' wishes – this clearly shows that there are limits to advocacy. In reality, most advocacy is based on a system of compromise, in other words, there are times when patients will lead and times when nurses will gently nudge them in another direction.

When counselling patients, it is so important to be clear about the limits of advocacy; failure to do this may compromise the patient's trust and any hope of a therapeutic relationship. Commenting upon the precarious nature of the themes surrounding patient advocacy, Kendrick (1994: 829) states:

> When patients realise their best interests are not represented as a mirror of their own wishes, it can conflict with the trust placed in the health care team. What emerges from this is the realisation that care which was supposed to be delivered with a velvet glove carries with it a fist of steel.

ASSESSMENT ACTIVITY

Consider the structure in this chapter and reflect on the following points:
- How do you feel about structuring counselling? Is it always necessary?
- What are the pros and cons of structure in the counselling relationship?
- What is it about structure that could be ethically objectionable?
- How have you structured conversations with patients up to this point?
- How do you evaluate what you do with patients, after you have talked to them?
- Do you think you are suitably placed to act as the patient's advocate?

Conclusion

This chapter has considered the issue of *structure* in the counselling relationship in nursing. It has been argued that there are a number of advantages in structuring in this way. It has been noted that nurses are mostly under some sort of *time* pressure and that structuring the relationship can make it easier to manage the time element of the relationship. The chapter has also raised questions about the degree to which the nurse counselling should *lead* the client in a counselling conversation. Finally, this chapter has also examined the relationship between advocacy and counselling.

5 COUNSELLING SKILLS 1: LISTENING AND ATTENDING

CHAPTER AIMS

- **To explore the concept of listening**
- **To consider the behavioural aspects of listening**
- **To explore ways of becoming a better listener**

Introduction

In Chapter 1, we discovered that listening is probably the most important part of counselling. In the end, it is not what we say to people, it is how we listen to them. Listening involves a range of qualities and activities. First, it requires that we see the other person as *important*. We are prepared to give this other person our time. Second, it requires that we are *interested* in the other person. We cannot listen if we are bored by what we hear. Third, we must be prepared to *work* at listening. Most of us are not born good listeners. We have to put in the effort to become better. Fourth, we must be able to separate the problems of other people from our own problems. What another person tells us about himself or herself does not necessarily relate to *us*. We do not have to assume that what people tell us *affects* us. We must learn, perhaps, to distinguish between another person's problems and our own. If we do not do this, we will find that we confuse ourselves and we fail to listen carefully. Listening, then, is a curious combination of giving our complete attention to another person and also of being able to detach ourselves a little from the other person.

Listening and attending

To listen to another person is the most human of actions. In counselling, it is the crucial skill. The experiential exercises that follow aim to develop the skill of listening and giving attention. Listening refers to the process of *hearing* what the client is saying. Hearing encompasses not only the words that are being used but also the non-verbal aspects of the encounter. Thus, *attending* refers to the counsellor's skill in paying attention to the client – in keeping attention focused 'out' as described in the first chapter.

Hargie *et al.* (1981) list the general functions of listening as follows:

- to focus specifically upon the messages being communicated by the other person;
- to gain full, accurate understanding of the other person's communication;
- to convey interest, concern and attention;
- to encourage full, open and honest expression;
- to develop an 'other-centred' approach during an interaction.

It is vital that the person *notices*: notices their own feelings and thoughts, their own body position, posture, eye contact and so forth. The mystic George Gurdjieff maintained that for most of what we call the waking state, we were, in fact, 'asleep' – we simply did not *notice* (Reyner 1984). Ouspensky, a follower of Gurdjieff, went on to suggest that we only really learned new things and remembered what had happened to us when we 'stayed awake'. The Christian mystic Simone Weil added a spiritual dimension to the notion of attending when she suggested that true noticing of what was happening around us was an acknowledgment of God (Weil 1967). Brother Lawrence called noticing and attending 'The Practice of the Presence of God' (Lawrence 1981). Thus, the topic has been addressed from both secular and spiritual points of view.

Listening behaviours

Gerard Egan (1986) offered an acronym for recalling the important aspects of non-verbal activity during the listening process. Egan suggested that, in Western countries, these behaviours are associated with effective listening. The acronym that Egan offers is as follows:

S. Sit squarely in relation to the client
O. Maintain an open position
L. Lean slightly forward
E. Maintain comfortable eye contact with the client
R. Relax while listening.

Sitting squarely means sitting opposite the person who is being listened to, rather than next to them. In this way, the one doing the listening can see *all* of the other person and can observe the non-verbal behaviours of the talker. The position also demonstrates interest in the other person.

An open position means that the listener does not have his or her arms crossed. Such crossings can create real or psychological barriers. The *closed* position can often be construed as being defensive, as we shall see in the next exercise.

Eye contact should be steady and appropriate. No one wants to be stared at but neither do they want to feel that the person who is supposed to be listening to them will look anywhere but at them. As we have noted, cultural factors, too, play a part in determining how much or how little eye contact may be made. Eye contact may also depend upon the relative status of the pair involved. Finally, the listener should try to sit quietly and be relaxed. When listening to another person, we do not have to be constantly rehearsing what *we* will say next. Nor do we have to relate everything that is said to *us* and to our own thoughts and feelings.

Egan's guidelines on how to sit when listening to another person may be useful as a baseline. Clearly, no one wants to talk to a person who sits and looks like a statue! On the other hand, it does not help very much to sit, lounge and fidget when listening. The SOLER acronym serves as a gentle reminder and guide whilst listening and counselling.

There is a danger, if these sorts of behaviours are adhered to *too* literally, that the client will *notice* the 'forced' behaviour of the counsellor. These sorts of behaviours are useful if they become 'natural' to the user but less so if the user feels uncomfortable with them. One of the authors (P.B.) is reminded of when he first trained as a counsellor. Shortly afterwards, he was talking to a friend, who wanted to talk through some problems. After a short period, the friend said 'I've just realised that I'm being counselled!'

Hargie *et al.* (1994) offer the following basic guidelines to be borne in mind when listening:

- Get physically prepared to listen.
- Be mentally prepared to listen objectively.
- Use spare thought time positively.
- Avoid interrupting the speaker where possible.
- Organise the speaker's messages into appropriate categories and, where possible, into chronological order.
- Don't overuse blocking tactics.
- Remember that listening is hard work.

Towards more effective listening

It is a fact that we have to work at listening. However, Woolf *et al.* (1983) offer some useful pointers to what we can do to facilitate effective listening. Their ten points are as follows:

1. Do not stereotype the speaker.
2. Avoid distractions.
3. Arrange a conducive environment (adequate ventilation, lighting, seating, etc.).
4. Be psychologically prepared to listen.
5. Keep an open, analytical mind, searching for the central thrust of the speaker's message.
6. Identify supporting arguments and facts.
7. Do not dwell on one or two aspects at the expense of others.
8. Delay judgement or refutation, until you have heard the entire message.
9. Do not formulate your next question while the speaker is relating information.
10. Be objective.

Definitions

Listening is the act of forgetting one's self and giving full and caring attention to another person. It involves an unjudgemental quality and an ability to be 'free floating' in one's attention to the other person. For here is a paradox: if we listen *too* closely to *everything* that another person says, we are likely to lose the 'drift' of what they are saying. We need to keep a *general* attention to the totality of what they are saying, whilst keeping an eye out for the important details.

DIALOGUE 5.1

Consider the following dialogue between a nurse and a patient. Consider the ways in which the nurse does and does not demonstrate that she is listening, carefully to what the patient is saying.

'How are you feeling?'

'My stomach hurts.'

'It's bound to – you've had an operation.'

'Yes, but, inside, it feels uncomfortable. I've had it before. I get a bit sick, sometimes, at home, and it feels like that, really.'

'It's probably bruising. That happens after an operation on your stomach.'

'My wife will be bringing me in something.'

'Oh, you can't take any medication other than the things that the doctor has prescribed.'

'Not, this is sort of a mixture. Fruit juice and things.'

'You mustn't just take any medication . . .'

'I wonder what it is?'

'What?'

'The stomach. It's funny at the moment. I feel sort of upset.'

'Don't worry so much. You'll be all right.'

'Thanks, nurse. I'll call you if I need anything.'

QUESTIONS ABOUT THE DIALOGUE

Give some consideration to the *two worlds* of the client and the nurse. The nurse, perhaps, is used to thinking about operations and about 'stomachs' in certain ways. The language and the way that he talks suggests that the client may be talking about quite different things. As a result, the nurse and the client are not really 'connecting'.

■ What could have helped the nurse to understand what the client was trying to say?

■ How would *you* have handled this conversation?

■ Was the nurse *listening*?

■ What were the *indicators* that suggest that she was or was not really listening?

REFLECTIONS

'Are you listening to me?' – Have you ever been asked that question? It may be that you really were listening but something about your manner gave the impression that your attention was elsewhere. This perception could have been caused by a casual gaze at the clock, body language that seemed detached and uninterested or eye contact on anything other than the person who is talking to you. There are many reasons why people may think we are not listening and, on occasion, they will be right in their assumption. To really listen to someone is hard work. If you are tired or stressed, then it becomes increasingly difficult to give total attention to someone else.

As nurses, the ability to listen to patients is a skill that has to be developed and fine-tuned. If we do not listen to what patients tell us, we may miss vital hints and information that could effect care planning and delivery. Also, patients who feel they are not being listened to may be reluctant to place their trust in the health care team. Once this happens, the foundations for a therapeutic relationship are violated – after all, would you trust someone who did not listen to what you said? For these reasons, listening is the heart of communication.

In the previous dialogue, the nurse begins with an open question that invites the patient to share how he is feeling. The patient then gives a reply that all is not well: 'My stomach hurts'. This could have been explored by the nurse through a variety of questions, for example:

■ 'Can you tell me where the "hurt" is exactly?'

■ 'How long have you had it for?'

■ 'Do you find that certain positions make it better or worse?'

■ Have you experienced this ever before?

Instead of inviting the patient to talk, the nurse gives a closed response with the stock answer 'It's bound to – you've had an operation'. The patient then offers some vital clues about the nature and history of the problem:

'Yes, but, inside, it feels uncomfortable. I've had it before. I get a bit sick, sometimes, at home, and it feels like that, really.'

This tells the nurse:

■ The man has an 'uncomfortable' sensation rather than pain.

- The sensation is accompanied by feelings of nausea.
- It has happened before, at home.

Sometimes, as nurses, we can become conditioned to react in certain ways by the clinical environment in which we work. The patient has had an abdominal operation and the nurse is 'blinkered' by viewing his responses purely within the confines of someone who has had surgery. In doing this, the patient is denied care that mirrors his unique and individual needs. The man has offered vital information, but the nurse is rigidly fixed into seeing him in a postoperative context and gives a response that shows she has not listened to anything he has said:

> 'It's probably bruising. That happens after an operation on your stomach.'

It would have been more appropriate for the nurse to ask the following sort of questions:

- Are there any particular things that make this feeling of discomfort worse or better?
- Does this uncomfortable sensation feel like 'butterflies' in the stomach?
- Do you ever wake up with the sensation in the middle of the night or first thing in the morning?
- Do you take any medication for it and does this relieve the feeling?
- The nurse could also gently enquire whether or not the man is constipated.

By not being focused on what the man is saying, the nurse loses a vibrant opportunity to understand the meaning, history and context of the 'uncomfortable' feeling in his stomach.

The patient begins to realise that the nurse is not listening to his explanation and complaint about the 'uncomfortable' feeling; he resorts to 'home comforts' and says 'My wife will be bringing me in something'. This, in itself, reflects poorly on the nurse's lack of listening skills – it is poor practice when a patient in hospital has to seek solace from home for abdominal discomfort. Even then, the nurse is completely fixed into surgical mode and automatically thinks that this means medication that may conflict with what he is receiving in hospital:

> 'Oh, you can't take any medication other than the things that the doctor has prescribed.'

After reassuring the nurse that his wife will bring in nothing more threatening than a concoction of fruit juices, the patient still tries to focus the nurse's attention on the uncomfortable feeling in his stomach:

> 'I wonder what it is?'
> 'What?'
> 'The stomach. It's funny at the moment. I feel sort of upset.'

By saying that he feels 'sort of upset', the man is giving a clear indication that the uncomfortable feeling is concerned with some sort of anxiety. Admitting vulnerability and fear is never easy, and when patients pluck up the courage to be open about their fears they should be gently encouraged not brusquely dismissed. The thing which is troubling this patient may have been completely unrelated to his abdominal surgery. The nurse will never know what the root of the problem is because the patient's search for a listening ear is dismissed with: 'Don't worry so much. You'll be all right.'

Ultimately, the patient becomes resigned to the fact the nurse is not going to address his problem and he says: 'Thanks, nurse. I'll call you if I need anything.' The truth is that the patient will probably be reluctant to seek that nurse's help ever again.

The nurse in this dialogue did not listen to anything the patient was saying. All that she heard was received at a very superficial level that left the patient feeling completely unheeded. The point is that the patient cast down some jewels of information that related greatly to his care and treatment in hospital. By not listening, the nurse denied the patient access to fuller, more vibrant and individualised care.

ASSESSMENT ACTIVITY BOX

Read through this chapter again and consider the following questions:

- To what degree could *your* listening skills be improved?
- Who do you know who exemplifies, for you, excellent listening skills?
- Why is listening so important?

Conclusion

This chapter has considered the idea that *listening* is the basis of effective counselling. By listening to another person, we are better placed to enter their *perceptual world* – the way in which they view their own and other people's worlds. We cannot assume that everyone sees the world the way that we do. Nor can we assume that everyone uses *language* in the way that we do. This confusion over language can lead to misunderstandings. In the example illustrated in this chapter, if the nurse had taken a little time to explore what the patient meant by 'stomach' and what he meant by feeling 'uncomfortable' in that region, she may have been better placed to help him.

6 COUNSELLING SKILLS 2: A COUNSELLING SKILLS TOOL-KIT

CHAPTER AIMS

- **To identify some of the skills of counselling**
- **To explore further ways of learning counselling skills**

Introduction

The previous chapter identified that listening was the basis of effective counselling. However, it cannot *only* involve listening: there must be some *talking* involved! The degree and type of talking will depend, largely, on the theoretical orientation of the counsellor. We have already alluded to the *client-centred* approach to counselling and in this chapter we will look at it more closely. We will also note that there are more *prescriptive* and *confrontational* approaches.

The client-centred approach to counselling

The client-centred approach to counselling was developed by the American psychologist and humanistic psychotherapist, Carl Rogers. During the first part of his career, he used an approach that he called *educational therapy*, which was quite different to the client-centred approach. He believed, during his period of using the educational approach, that the best way to help parents with 'problem' children was to give those parents appropriate and up-to-date information about child psychology in order to enable them to make decisions about how they should act. Like many people at that time, he believed that information giving could affect people's behaviour. He found, however, that

his form of therapy did not work and changed, radically, in his practice. Over the years (spanning from the late 1930s to the 1980s), he developed the idea of the client-centred approach, which, later, he developed further into *student-centred learning*.

Essential to the client-centred approach is that the individual, as a fully functioning person, can both find solutions to his or her problems and work through towards problem resolution – and without their being given advice by another person. This form of counselling depends upon two things. First, the counsellor has to hold the view that people have a dynamic tendency to 'grow' if given the time and space. Second, the counsellor has to resist any temptation to 'fix things' for the client. In Rogers' formulation of the client-centred approach, the client can *always* be trusted to find his or her own solutions.

The philosophical background to this approach may be found in existentialism (the philosophy that suggests that people are ultimately and in every way responsible for what they do) and in phenomenology (the study of individuals' views of the world). Client-centred counselling is concerned with helping people to find their own way through their problems, from the stage of *identifying* the problems to, eventually, solving them. Rogers (1951) summed up his approach to counselling in the following way:

- Counselling is concerned with a humanistic approach to helping by increasing self understanding, awareness and the expression of feeling.

- Counselling is non-directive and seeks to encourage the client to formulate his or her own awareness of the pattern of his or her life and experience in his or her own way, the therapist adopting an accepting, non-critical attitude and helping by reflecting the client's own responses.
- The client does not react to reality as others see it but to his or her own perceptions of reality. No person can know the client's thoughts and feelings as well as the client himself or herself, the client's own internal frame of reference being the best context in which to understand his or her behaviour. In order to understand others, it is necessary to know more about the self and vice versa.
- Each human being has within themselves the skills and capability to change his or her life and rectify his or her own problems.

Rogers' concept of an 'internal frame of reference' is a useful one in understanding the idea that each of us views the world from a slightly different or very different point of view. To develop Rogers' idea, it is as though we are seeing the world through a window (or frame) and as if that window not only restricts what we see in the world but also colours what we see. The personal construct psychologist George Kelly has elaborated this idea further by suggesting that each of us wears a pair of 'goggles' and those goggles affect the way we see the world. Sometimes, we have two or three pairs of goggles and are able to see things in different ways but, often, we return to the safety of the first pair. One of the tasks of the counsellor is to try to imagine what the world looks like through the client's window or goggles. This is not a particularly easy task, but an important one. The process can also be personally rewarding. We can begin to change our own 'windows' or 'goggles' and begin to see the world differently, ourselves. Rogers wrote of an 'expanding frame of reference' in counselling, suggesting that as the client and counsellor talk, so each of their frames of reference develop to take in more and more aspects of the world and to see the world in various ways.

The term 'world', in this context, may be taken to include *everything* that is going on about us. The term is not restricted in any way to the physical world. In this way, the patient's world includes not only the physical environment but also the people in it, the network of relationships, the attitudes that

he or she has, the ways that he or she has of thinking and feeling about things, and so on.

Rogers also suggested that certain *personal qualities* of the counsellor contribute to making the counselling relationship therapeutic. He claimed that the following qualities were both *necessary* and *sufficient* for therapeutic change to occur. Three clusters of personal qualities were identified:

1. warmth and genuineness
2. empathic understanding
3. unconditional positive regard.

The three clusters of qualities are now briefly described and related to nursing.

WARMTH AND GENUINENESS

Warmth, in the nursing relationship, refers to being approachable and open to the patient or colleague. Schulman (1982) argues that the following characteristics are involved in demonstrating the concept of warmth: equal worth, absence of blame, non-defensiveness and closeness. Warmth is as much a frame of mind as a skill and perhaps one developed through being honest with yourself and being prepared to be open with others. It also involves treating the other person as an equal human being.

Martin Buber (1958), the philosopher and therapist, made a distinction between the 'I–it' relationship and the 'I–thou (or 'I–you') relationship. In the I–it relationship, one person treats the other as an object, as a thing. In the I–thou relationship, there occurs a meeting of persons, transcending any differences there may be in terms of status, background, lifestyle, belief or value systems. In the I–thou relationship, there is a sense sharing and of mutuality, a sense that can be contagious and is of particular value in nursing.

Thus, warmth must be offered by the nurse but the feeling may not necessarily be reciprocated by the client. There is, as well, another problem with the notion of warmth. We all perceive personal qualities in different sorts of ways. One person's warmth is another person's sickliness or sentimentality. We cannot guarantee how our 'warmth' will be perceived by the other person. In a more general way, however, 'warmth' may be compared with 'coldness'. It is clear that the 'cold' person would not be the ideal person to undertake helping another person in a nursing setting! It is salutary, however, to reflect on the degree to which there are 'cold' people working in the nursing arena and to question why this may be so. It is possible that interpersonal skills training may help this situation for it may be that some 'cold' people are unaware of their coldness.

To a degree, however, our relationships with others tend to be self-monitoring. To a degree, we anticipate, as we go on with a relationship, the effect we are having on others and modify our presentation of self accordingly. Thus, we soon get to know if our 'warmth' is too much for the patient or colleague or is being perceived by him or her in a negative way. This ability to constantly monitor ourselves and our relationships is an important part of the process of developing interpersonal and counselling skills.

Genuineness, too, is another important aspect of the relationship. In one sense, the issue is black or white. We either genuinely care for the person in front of us or we do not. We cannot easily fake professional interest. We must *be* interested. Some people, however, will interest us more than others. Often, those clients who remind us of our own problems or our own personalities will interest us most of all. This is not so important as our having a genuine interest in the fact that the relationship is happening at all.

On the surface of it, there may appear to be a conflict between the concept of genuineness and the self-monitoring alluded to above. Self-monitoring may be thought of as 'artificial' or contrived and therefore not genuine. The 'genuineness' discussed here relates to the nursing professional's interest in the human relationship that is developing between the two people. Any ways in which that relationship can be enhanced must serve a valuable purpose. It is quite possible to be 'genuine' and yet be aware of what is happening – genuine and yet committed to increasing interpersonal competence.

EMPATHIC UNDERSTANDING

Empathy is different to sympathy. Sympathy suggests 'feeling sorry' for the other person or, perhaps, identifying with how they feel. If a person sympathises, they imagine themselves as being in the other person's position. With empathy, the person tries to imagine how it is to be the other person. Feeling sorry for that person does not really come into it. Being empathic, says Rogers (1967),

> means entering the private perceptual world of the other and becoming thoroughly at home in it. It involves being sensitive,

moment to moment, to the changing felt meanings which flow in this other person, to the fear or rage or tenderness or confusion or whatever.

The process of developing empathy involves something of an act of faith. When we empathise with another person, we cannot know what the outcome of that empathising will be. If we pre-empt the outcome of our empathising, we are already not empathising – we are thinking of solutions and of ways of influencing the client towards a particular goal that we have in mind. The process of empathising involves entering into the perceptual world of the other person, without necessarily knowing where that process will lead to.

Developing empathic understanding is the process of exploring the client's world, with the client, neither judging nor necessarily offering advice. Perhaps it can be achieved best through the process of carefully attending and listening to the other person and, perhaps, by use of the skills known as 'reflection', which is discussed in Chapter 8 of this book. It is also a 'way of being', a disposition towards the client, a willingness to explore the other person's problems and to allow the other person to express themselves fully. Again, as with all aspects of the 'client-centred' approach to caring, the empathic approach is underpinned by the idea that it is the client, in the end, who will find their own way through and will find their own answers to their problems in living. To be empathic is to be a fellow traveller, a friend to the person as they undertake the search. Empathic understanding, then, invokes the notion of 'befriending'.

There are, of course, limitations to the degree to which we can truly empathise. Because we all live in different 'worlds' based on our particular culture, education, physiology, belief systems and so forth, we all view that world slightly differently. Thus, to truly empathise with another person would involve actually becoming that other person! We can, however, strive to get as close to the perceptual world of the other by listening and attending and by suspending judgement. We can also learn to forget ourselves, temporarily, and to give ourselves as completely as we can to the other person. There is an interesting paradox involved here. First, we need self-awareness to enable us to develop empathy. Then we need to forget ourselves in order to give, truly, our empathic attention to the other person.

UNCONDITIONAL POSITIVE REGARD

Carl Rogers' phrase 'unconditional positive regard' (Rogers 1967) conveys a particularly important predisposition towards the client, by the nurse. Rogers also called it 'prizing' or even just 'accepting'. It means that the client is viewed with dignity and valued as a worthwhile and positive human being. The 'unconditional' prefix refers to the idea that such regard is offered without any preconditions. Often, in relationships, some sort of reciprocity is demanded: I will like you (or love you) as long as you return that liking or loving. Rogers is asking that the feelings that the nursing professional holds for the client should be undemanding and not require reciprocation.

There is a suggestion of an inherent 'goodness' within the client, bound up in Rogers' notion of unconditional positive regard. This notion of persons as essentially good can be traced back, at least to Rousseau's 'Emile', and is philosophically problematic. Arguably, notions such as 'goodness' and 'badness' are social constructions and to argue that a person is born good or bad is fraught with difficulties. However, as a practical starting point in the nursing relationship, it seems to be a good idea that we assume an inherent, positive and life-asserting characteristic in the client. It seems difficult to argue otherwise. It would be odd, for instance, to engage in the process of counselling with the view that the person was essentially bad, negative and unlikely to grow or develop!

Unconditional positive regard, then, involves a deep and positive feeling for the other person, perhaps equivalent, in the health professions, to what Alistair Campbell has called 'moderated love' (Campbell 1984a). He talks of 'lovers and professors', suggesting that certain professionals profess to love – thus, claiming both the ability to be professional and to express altruistic love or disinterested love for others. It is interesting that Campbell seems to be suggesting that a nursing professional can 'professionally care for' or even 'professionally love' his or her client.

This, then, is a short sketch of the client-centred approach to counselling and the personal qualities required of client-centred counselling. It is important to note that not *all* counselling is of this sort. It is fairly clear that there are a number of counselling agencies based on *information giving*. If, for instance, you wanted AIDS counselling, you would expect to be given up-to-date and sensitive information about how the AIDS virus is transmitted and on

how to avoid contacting it. Clearly, in these circumstances, the client-centred approach would be inadequate.

The other point is that the client-centred approach to counselling takes *time* (as well as an ultimate optimism in people's ability to change for the better). We might argue that there is room for something of a compromise here. First, most nurses have a considerable amount of life experience – this will be more true, presumably, of older nurses, but it may well be true of younger ones, too. Second, many of the counselling conversations that nurses have with patients *will* involve the passing on of information. It is important that such information *does* get passed on and it is not sufficient merely to wait until patients ask for it. Therefore, our argument here is that nurses who counsel patients will probably be wise to combine some of the elements of the client-centred approach with information giving.

There is another, practical way of looking at this. We might say that *personal and emotional* problems might best be dealt with by the client-centred approach. On the other hand, *medical and nursing* problems might involve a more prescriptive, information-giving approach. Let us consider, for example, the person who is recovering from a myocardial infarct. Such a person will have a range of problems. First, he is likely to be very anxious about a range of things. Will he have another heart attack? If so, is it likely to be fatal? Will his lifestyle have to change dramatically? Is he getting old and 'past it'? Will he be able to exercise? Will he be able to have sexual relations with his partner? Will he get over the anxiety he feels at the moment? Will his family accept him as he is? Questions like these cannot, of course, be neatly divided into 'personal' and 'medical' categories, but the general principles of helping by using a mixture of the client-centred and information-giving approaches are likely to be useful. No one, presumably, would rely purely on the client-centred approach to dealing with this man's anxieties, but neither would they rely only on giving him information. As in many things, the 'middle path' seems a good one to take.

Certainly, there is evidence that *information giving* is an important part of the health care professional's skill. Ley (1982) offered the following evidence in support of effective information giving:

- Between 66 and 93% of patients approved of being told they had cancer or were terminally ill.
- There is no increase in distress as a result of extra information about test results or access to case notes.

- There is no reduction in compliance or increased side-effects with fuller information about drugs. On the contrary, as predictable from psychological theories ... there is evidence of increased emotional disturbance where information is inadequate.

Types of counselling intervention

There are a variety of things that clients can say during counselling conversations and they will now be described. The list of *general* counselling interventions is as follows:

- questions
- reflections
- empathy-developing statements
- checks for understanding
- explaining.

QUESTIONS

Questions can be broadly divided into *open* and *closed* types. Open questions are one to which the asker does not really know the answer. They allow the talker to 'open up' and be more expansive. Examples of open questions include 'How do you feel about that?', 'What did you do?', 'What are your plans?' As a rule, open questions are useful in counselling. Closed questions are ones that have a specific and often short answer to them. Examples of closed questions are 'What is your name?', 'Are you in pain?', 'Have you completed the course of tablets?' Closed questions are useful as part of an information-gathering interview but not, generally, so useful in counselling – except where a piece of information is sought.

Dickson *et al.* (1989) offer a useful summary of the purposes of questions, as follows:

- to obtain precise information from patients
- to open interactions (e.g. 'How are you today?')
- to diagnose particular difficulties which patients may be experiencing
- to focus attention upon a specific area
- to assess the patient's condition and their knowledge and understanding of it
- to maintain control of the interaction
- to encourage maximum participation from patients
- to demonstrate an interest in the patient

- to help create enlightenment (e.g. 'Did you know that ... ?')
- to facilitate the discussion of attitudes and feelings.

REFLECTIONS

Reflections are the means by which the counsellor encourages the client to say more, to continue on a particular track. The following is an example of a nurse using reflection.

'I felt worse for a time, much worse. I didn't know what to do ... '
'You didn't know what to do ... '

'I was on my own. There was nobody I could talk to. There are a number of points that need to be made about reflection. First, the nurse's reflection should not become a *question*. If it does become a question, the following situation can occur, which hardly moves the conversation on:

'I feel uncomfortable at the moment. I'm not sure what to do ... '
'You're not sure what to do?'
'No.' (!)

The counsellor should aim at feeding back the reflection in much the same *tone of voice* as the one in which it was delivered by the client.

Second, reflection should be used cautiously. So much has been written about reflection as a counselling activity that it has become something of a cliché. Overuse of it can seem intrusive. However, skilled use of it can ensure that the client stays on track and develops his or her line of thinking, and it is not intrusive.

EMPATHY DEVELOPING STATEMENTS

Empathy-developing statements are ones where the counsellor makes a considered guess at the feelings behind what the client is saying and conveys this to the client. Examples of empathy developing statements include 'It sounds as though you were very uncomfortable. ...', 'You sound quite sad at the moment...', 'You must have enjoyed that...'

Various ways of expressing empathy have been enumerated by French (1993) as follows:

- By identifying themes i.e. by tentatively suggesting thoughts or trends that run like continuous threads through the previous conversations. For example, one may say, 'This idea of loneliness seems to have been mentioned several times, is this a major concern?'

- Helping the client to come to the ultimate conclusions of what has been said, i.e. 'What do you think would happen if you cannot persuade John to go to school?'
- By pointing to possible bridges or links between seemingly unrelated issues, facts or feelings, i.e. 'Do you see any way in which your comment about disliking authority is linked to your relationship with Sister Bleweit?'
- Stating clearly things that the client may have said in vague, disjointed or confused terms, for example:

> P: 'I'm not sure about this operation. It seems ... well, silly to have it, but it's for my own sake, so they say. ... But I'm not convinced. ... It doesn't look as if I have any alternative although I suppose we all have the right to make up our own minds.'
>
> N: 'It seems as though you are saying that you do not want to have the operation? *or* I can sense that you feel pressurised into having the operation.'

CHECKS FOR UNDERSTANDING

Checks for understanding are useful when the nurse wants to make sure that what the client says is completely clear. Examples of such checks include: 'Let me just go over that again. You said ...', 'Can I just check something with you? You said ...'

It should be emphasised, though, that the things people say and the skills they use in framing sentences are probably not nearly as important as the general approach they have towards the client. The best counselling is not something in which the counsellor is constantly paying attention to the phrasing of interventions. Rather, it is a particularly sensitive way of 'being with' the client or patient and paying attention to how that other person views the world.

EXPLAINING

There will be many times in which nurses have to explain details or procedures to patients and clients, both within and outside of the counselling relationship. The notion of 'explaining' fits into the 'information-giving' approach to counselling. Dickson *et al.* (1989) suggest that, depending on the context, the purposes of explaining are to:

- provide information
- simplify complexities
- correct mistaken beliefs
- give advice
- aid patient compliance
- highlight the important elements of any procedure
- offer reassurance and reduce uncertainty
- justify one's actions and recommendations
- increase patient satisfaction
- ensure patient understanding.

French (1993) offers a useful set of pointers about explaining things to patients before anything happens to them. In nursing, much attention is given to the need to reassure patients prior to procedures, and French's points formalise this reassurance and make it more operational. He suggests that at the beginning of an encounter with a patient it is important to do the following:

- Tell the patient what she is going to do and what is going to happen.
- Give reasons why any information being sought is necessary.
- Ask if the patient has any misgivings, and answer any questions by providing a full explanation.
- Advise the patient what he has to do and what is expected of him.
- Check the accuracy of any information already collected, where appropriate.
- Gain the attention and co-operation of the patient.

On the other hand, Frost notes that reassurance, as an aspect of explaining, is not limited only to words. Frost (1974) suggests that:

> Reassurance does not necessarily mean words; actions are not always imperative either. It is sufficient that a nurse can cope with her own emotions well enough to enable her to sit quietly and without tension while the patient is struggling to formulate her thoughts. ... Anyone can hand out advice, but it is the intelligent nurse who knows how to convey serenity and acceptance without saying one word.

Frost describes something very important here. It is the ability to sit quietly and just to 'be' with the client. Often, when we are worried about another person's situation, we are tempted to 'overtalk', to fill silences, and we feel that we must come up with some answers. As Frost points out, often, the most therapeutic thing that we can offer another person is our quiet – sometimes silent – presence.

Definitions

Listening remains the basic ingredient of all good counselling. However, counsellors and clients also *talk*. The 'counsellor talk' will depend on the style of counselling undertaken. The *client-centred* approach to counselling argues that people are free to determine their own futures and, given the time and space, will make the 'right' decisions for themselves, if they are allowed to identify and solve their own problems. It has been noted that, in nursing, there are times when information giving is likely to be both appropriate and necessary.

DIALOGUE 6.1

Read the following dialogue *critically* and identify the times at which the counsellor seems to be using a *client-centred* approach (which encourages self-directed decision making and when she uses a more *directive* or information-giving approach. Note, too, when the counselling interventions are just not very good!

'So, when did you first go into hospital?'
'When I was twelve. I had loads of operations on my leg. They broke it in about ten places.'
'I doubt whether they really did that!'
'They did! The doctor told me that they had to!'
'Well, don't let's worry about that. How are you coping now?'
'All right. I can get to work on most days but sometimes my leg hurts so much that I can't.'
'What do you do on days like that?'
'I phone up and tell them that I won't be in. They know about my leg and they are very understanding.'
'So it's working out well? They support you?'
'Yes, very much. They're very good to me.'
'They obviously appreciate your work.'
'They seem to. I got a bonus last Christmas. And, anyway, I like it there.'
'What do you do about exercise?'
'Not a lot. I'm putting on weight.'
'What do you feel about that?'

'I should lose some, I suppose. What do you think?'
'Well, sometimes it's just a question of eating the right things. Diets aren't really a good idea. You may want to keep an eye on your weight. If you put on too much, it can be a strain on your joints.'
'I eat a lot of junk food!'
'*Could* you eat 'proper' food?'
'Oh yes. I've just got a bit lazy.'
'Do you think you could start a healthy eating programme?'
'Eating programme. Do you mean "*proper eating*"?'
'Yes – I suppose. (Laughs)'
'Well, I'll just have to make sure that I get to the supermarket twice a week.'
'And you could walk there?'
'I could. That would give me some exercise.'
'It would be a start. A good start.'

QUESTIONS ABOUT THE DIALOGUE

- To what degree did the nurse use client-centred interventions?
- What sort of *information giving* did she engage in and was her information accurate?
- How would you have handled this conversation?
- In what way could the conversation be continued?
- What would be the key issues in such a continuation?

REFLECTIONS

The essential theme in the client-centred approach is that the person being counselled has freedom to be self-directing about any decisions that are made. This reflects a central principle with client-centredness, namely, that people have a dynamic tendency to 'grow', given the necessary time and space. At times in the previous dialogue, the nurse uses this approach coupled with, sometimes, a more directive manner. We will shortly analyse the dialogue to see at which times each of these approaches were used. However, another important requisite for counselling, of any sort, is trust, and this seems to be placed on a precarious footing right from the start of the dialogue.

The discussion starts with the patient responding to the nurse's open and client-centred enquiry about the first admission to hospital:

'When I was twelve. I had loads of operations on my leg. They broke it in about ten places.'

This is the patient's opening gambit and is given as an honest response to an open question; yet the nurse immediately questions the validity of the claim:

'I doubt whether they really did that!'

There is no need to doubt the patient's response, yet as soon as such language is introduced into the conversation, it makes the patient become defensive. This may have the effect of making the patient think that the nurse does not believe what is being said. Moreover, it can also make the patient think that everything else that is said will be taken with a 'pinch of salt'; this confronts the essential themes of honesty and trust on which so such much of the patient–nurse association intrinsically relies, as Bok (1978: 36) eloquently affirms: 'Veracity (*truthfulness*) is the cornerstone of relationships among human beings'.

After the nurse's expression of doubt, the patient affirms his position:

'They did! The doctor told me that they had to!'

However, the nurse is still reluctant to accept the patient's word and dismisses this part of their conversation; the nurse then moves the dialogue to reflect a more positive client-centred approach:

'Well, don't let's worry about that. How are you coping now?'

There was nothing to stop the nurse accepting what the patient had said as the truth. To introduce doubt breeds mistrust and this opening part of the dialogue does not mirror good practice. However, by asking 'How are you coping now?' the nurse offers the patient the oportunity to focus on the problem and share how it impinges on everyday life:

'All right. I can get to work on most days but sometimes my leg hurts so much that I can't.'

The nurse then asks the client-centred question 'What do you do on days like that?' This asks the patient to explain how the problem is challenged in relation to work:

'I phone up and tell them that I won't be in. They know about my leg and they are very understanding.'

The nurse then asks a number of client-centred questions that reveal the patient's work situation to be rewarding in terms of both financial rewards and job satisfaction; the patient responds to the nurse's enquiry about being appreciated by colleagues:

'They seem to. I got a bonus last Christmas. And, anyway, I like it there.'

The nurse then changes tack and the direction of the conversation by asking 'What do you do about exercise?'

The patient give a limited response and acknowledges that weight gain is a problem

'Not a lot. I'm putting on weight.'

What the nurse has not picked up is that the patient's exercise options may be limited by the physical problem with the leg. It may have been feasible here to ask if the patient had seen a physiotherapist about non-weight-bearing exercise. The nurse's next question is very client-centred:

'What do you feel about that?'

This question moves the conversion on and creates an arena where the patient feels able to seek the nurse's advice about weight loss.

'I should lose some, I suppose. What do you think?'

The next response from the nurse combines both client-centredness with directive, information giving:

'Well, sometimes it's just a question of eating the right things. Diets aren't really a good idea. You may want to keep an eye on your weight. If you put on too much, it can be a strain on your joints.'

This response is directive because it offers information about good eating habits and the strain that excess weight can put on the joints; however, it is also client-centred because it tells the patient: 'You may want to keep an eye on your weight' – this offers the patient freedom to decide about the issue of exercise and weight loss.

The next part of the dialogue is both humerous and important – humerous because the patient seems to tease the nurse about the use of the jargonistic term 'healthy eating programme':

'Do you think you think you could start a healthy eating programme?'
'Eating programme, do you mean "*proper eating*"?'
'Yes – I suppose. (laughs)

Humour is a vibrant and vital part of human relations and should be used whenever appropriate; it can inject energy into fraught situations and lift any occasion. A person usually has to feel safe before using humour (have you ever noticed how hard it is to tell a joke when you are nervous?); by making a funny comment the patient is showing ease with the situation. This opens the door for the patient to combine exercise with the purchase of healthy food – by walking to the supermarket a couple of times a week.

The conversation could then develop to form a plan to give the patient details about healthy eating and exercise. If the patient was agreeable, this could be combined with visits from the dietitian and physiotherapist prior to discharge. This illustrates how client-centred and directive approaches to counselling can create options and freedom of choice for the patient.

ASSESSMENT ACTIVITY BOX

Read through this chapter again and, in particular, review the section on client-centred counselling. Then consider the following questions:

- To what degree does the client-centred approach fit in with your own views about how counselling should be practised?
- What are the limitations of the client-centred approach?
- To what degree have you been practising this approach, already, in your nursing practice?

Conclusion

This chapter has offered a view of the ways in which the 'talking' part of counselling might be conducted. It has noted that the things counsellors say to clients will, to some degree, depend on their *approach* to counselling. The chapter has also described the client-centred approach to counselling and argued that such an approach might best be combined with *information giving* in nursing.

7 USING COUNSELLING SKILLS IN EVERYDAY LIFE

CHAPTER AIMS

- **To consider counselling as a 'natural' activity**
- **To explore everyday situations in which counselling skills might be used**

Introduction

Counselling is not an activity that is restricted to nursing and the caring or health care professions. It has wider application in the wider world. We counsel, in a sense, when we help out friends. We counsel when we talk to family members about their problems. However, we do not usually *label* such activity as counselling. And this is probably appropriate. It is probably true that no one, in everyday life – in families and in social circles – likes to be 'counselled' by other family members or friends.

On the other hand, we can learn a lot about how to counsel at work by observing ourselves in these more everyday settings. In a sense, the counselling approach must become a part of who we are. If counselling is to be effective in the professional context, we must learn to be 'full-time' helpers and carers. It should become part of the way we relate to people and not something that is 'turned on' when we go to work.

What are the ethical implications of all this? First, we might want to say that if we act in this way we are turning our families and friends into 'clients'. We can meet this argument from another point of view by saying that we do not have to think of *anyone* in terms of 'clients' and 'other people'. We simply relate to all people in helpful ways. This may sound a little 'Pollyanna-ish' and suggest that we should all go around with smiles on our faces, being pleasant to everyone we meet. Clearly, this cannot be the case. The point, though, is that we learn to *live* by listening to other people, by respecting their points of view, and so on.

None of this is to assume that we will not have 'off days'. We are all subject to moods and shifts of personality, depression, anxiety and other difficulties. However, if we are to become skilled counsellors, that ability to counsel must become incorporated into our way of being. Rogers, founding father of the client-centred approach, stressed the point that he felt least comfortable as a counsellor when he found himself using 'skills' and 'techniques'. Clearly, the philosophy and approach had become the man.

How, then, might we use counselling skills in everyday life – outside of the nursing profession. A short list of situations might include the following:

- when a friend is bereaved
- when a family member is experiencing relationship difficulties
- when there are interpersonal difficulties between you and another family member
- when talking to members of the public
- when talking to people in shops and offices
- when breaking good and bad news to other people.

Definitions

It is argued that in order to be a 'genuine' counsellor as well as a nurse, it is important to incorporate the various skills and attitudes of counselling into everyday life. This can be achieved by 'living' the approach and not by simply turning on counselling skills when going to work. It is acknowledged that this will not always be possible and that it is important to recognise 'off' periods.

DIALOGUE 7.1

'What do you think I should do? I've got a place at
   university but I really want to go to work now. I
   could get a job fairly easily – a couple of people
   have offered me jobs already.'
'What are the pros and cons of all this, then?'
'Don't know. I don't particularly want to go to university. I got sick of school, and university will just
   be more school. I really want to go to work.'
'Why are you questioning it, then?'
'Because I'm not sure, I suppose. You're right. If I
   really *didn't* want to go to university, at all, I
   wouldn't be thinking about it. I would just get a
   job.'
'So you do have some doubts.'
'I do. . . . Perhaps I should go to university and give
   it a try.'
'What, do the first year and see how you get on?'
'Something like that. What do you think?'
'If it was me, I would probably go to university. I
   would get a job *after* that.'
'Yes, but that's *you*, not me!'
'I know, but you *asked* me!'
'True! Sorry. I'll have to keep thinking about it. You
   may be right, though. I think, deep down, that I
   do want to go to university. All I've got to sort out,
   though, is whether or not I like the *idea* of going
   to university, rather than actually going . . . '

QUESTIONS ABOUT THE DIALOGUE

Read through the dialogue again and consider the
following questions:

- *Is* this counselling?
- What counselling principles might be being used
  here?
- When were counselling principles abandoned in
  the conversation?
- What was the effect?
- *Should* you attempt to counsel friends?

REFLECTIONS

We have already said that the skills of counselling
should be woven into the fabric of everyday life. It
would be extremely cold and clinical to 'switch'
into a caring, listening individual merely because
that fits in with the professional image of being a
nurse. What we can also say is that our ability to 'be
at one' with the needs of another human being is

strongly influenced by what is happening, at that
moment, in our own lives. If a person is worried,
troubled, tired and angst-ridden, it makes it very
difficult to be 'at one' with another person.

While acknowledging the limitations of being
human and how everyday trials confront and challenge us, making compassion and attentive listening part of our everyday life can embellish the way
we view the world and relate to others in it. We
may not use the term 'counselling' each time we
offer a listening ear to a friend, but using counselling skills may certainly help both parties to
focus on the problem at hand.

The previous dialogue could have taken place
anywhere and involves a dilemma that confronts
thousands of people every year – whether to go to
university or get a job:

> 'What do you think I should do? I've got a
> place at university but I really want to go to
> work now. I could get a job fairly easily – a
> couple of people have offered me jobs
> already.'

The response to this certainly mirrors a counselling
tradition; it is client-centred and asks for reflection:

> 'What are the pros and cons of all this, then?'

This challenges the person to think systematically
and carefully about the benefits or otherwise of
going to work or going to university. This clearly
has the desired effect of focusing the mind, as
shown by the person's response:

> 'Don't know. I don't particularly want to go to
> university. I got sick of school, and university
> will just be more school. I really want to go to
> work.'

The initial response of 'Don't know' suggests that
this is an area that has not been given a lot of
thought. However, being asked to think about the
'pros and cons' has galvanised the person to focus
on the issue. This shows dynamism and progress in
the conversation. The decision seems to have been
made that the person will go to work, an excellent
piece of questioning is then used that challenges the
whole basis of the conversation:

> 'Why are you questioning it, then?'

This asks the person to really search for the reasons
why they prefer to go to work rather than university. If the choice had already been made, what is
the point behind the conversation? The emphasis is
clearly being placed on the person to make the decision and not to rely on the person using counselling

skills for the answer. This serves to focus the person's mind on why the topic was brought into the conversation; this is mirrored in the response:

> 'Because I'm not sure, I suppose. You're right. If I really *didn't* want to go to university, at all, I wouldn't be thinking about it. I would just get a job.'

The person carries on with a client-centred approach that encourages reflection:

> 'So you do have some doubts.'

The person being counselled then shifts tack and offers the opinion that maybe university should be seen as an option to be tried:

> 'I do. . . . Perhaps I should go to university and give it a try.'

However, this, in effect, is where the counselling ends. The person offering counselling is asked:

> 'Something like that. What do you think?'

Instead of saying something like 'What I think isn't important; what is important is that you make a decision you feel comfortable with', the person offering counsel takes ownership of the question and gives an opinion that may influence the other person's ultimate decision:

> 'If it was me, I would probably go to university. I would get a job *after* that.'

This has the effect of throwing the conversation off course and the client-centred approach dissolves. The person affirms that the counsellor's opinion was not really requested – to which an inaccurate response is given:

> 'I know, but you *asked* me!'

The counsellor was not asked, and this then leads to a position where the other person apologises and asks a series of questions that show further areas of doubt. If the counsellor had remained focused, these issues may have arisen through the other person's reflections. As it is, what started as a conversation that had progression and real promise to solve a problem, ends with so many unchallenged and unexplored queries:

> 'True! Sorry. I'll have to keep thinking about it. You may be right, though. I think, deep down, that I *do* want to go to university. All I've got to sort out, though, is whether or not I like the *idea* of going to university, rather than actually going . . .'

This dialogue realistically reflects the sort of conversation that takes place between thousands of people up and down the country. If the person using counselling skills had been a little more focused, the scenario would have been brought to a much more productive conclusion.

So, should we counsel friends? The essential point is that we should not even think about doing so unless consent is given. We do not mean here a signed consent form, but the friend should certainly seek our counsel rather than us imposing it. For example, it would be folly to start counselling a recently bereaved friend who really just wanted time to 'be still' with the rawness of emotional turmoil. What could be offered is a silent presence or, if that is inappropriate, the offer that you are just a phone call away. To try and counsel people in an emotional quagmire, before they are ready, can have disastrous consequences – take the lead from them, do not try and lead them.

Counselling, then, when given as a response to welcoming consent, can embellish a friendship. The vital point to remember is that you must be sure you can stand the emotional intensity of counselling someone who is close to you. Failure to do this may compromise all those involved.

ASSESSMENT ACTIVITY BOX

Read through this chapter again and then consider the following questions:

- Do you think that there are major differences between counselling and talking to people at home?
- If so, is counselling really a *particular* activity at all? Or, is it just an elaboration of what we all do, all of the time?
- Should counselling skills be learned from training courses or from living life?

Conclusion

This chapter has discussed the idea of counselling as an activity that has to be *lived*. In the end, it is not merely a set of skills to be used in professional settings but an orientation towards people – an attitude to how people can be helped to help themselves. In this way, using counselling skills becomes a way of reflecting an empathic approach towards those we encounter in all aspects of everyday living.

8 PERSONAL DEVELOPMENT AND COUNSELLING

CHAPTER AIMS

- **To explore the concept of *personal development***
- **To identify ways in which nurses can become more self-aware**

Introduction

The person who works with people also has to work with himself or herself. The fact of hearing people talking about their problems and their life situations can be wearing. As we have seen, it can also make us call into question our own beliefs and values. And this is how it should be. No one should stop in their personal development. Life, in a way, is a continuous process of development and learning. The notion of 'lifelong learning' has been adopted by the English National Board for Nursing, Midwifery and Health Visiting and it sums up the philosophy exactly. No one has ever learned 'enough': we all have to continue our formal and informal education as we go through our careers and through life.

Values and beliefs clarification

Everyone holds values and beliefs and we cannot assume that we all hold the same ones. Anyone engaging in counselling, though, should examine their own values and beliefs for they always seep into the work that we do with clients. We cannot

easily *ignore* them but becoming aware of them can help us to appreciate when they are making a difference to what we do.

ACTIVITY BOX 8.1

Figure 8.1 is a questionnaire that is a method of exploring values and beliefs.

- Read through the questionnaire slowly and answer each item 'agree' or 'disagree'.
- As you do this, ask yourself the question 'Why?' This is, perhaps, the most important aspect of the exercise – identifying your reasons for holding the values and beliefs that you do.
- After you have worked through the questionnaire in Fig. 8.1, consider the one shown in Fig. 8.2.
- Again, circle the appropriate answer to each of the questions.

The aim of this part of the activity is to consider the degree to which you are influenced by your beliefs and values and the degree to which you feel they can or cannot be changed.

Beliefs and Values Questionnaire		
1. All nurses should learn counselling skills.	Agree	Disagree
2. Clients always know what is best for them.	Agree	Disagree
3. There is only one true religion.	Agree	Disagree
4. All religions have elements of truth in them.	Agree	Disagree
5. There should be heavier fines for drug abusers.	Agree	Disagree
6. The age of consent should be lowered.	Agree	Disagree
7. Cannabis should be legalised.	Agree	Disagree
8. Gay people should be allowed to marry.	Agree	Disagree
9. Most people are religious at some level.	Agree	Disagree
10. All nurses should be graduates.	Agree	Disagree
11. Nurse teachers should remain in clinical practice.	Agree	Disagree
12. The death penalty should be available for certain crimes.	Agree	Disagree
13. Those with mental health problems should not be allowed to vote.	Agree	Disagree
14. Most people would benefit from counselling.	Agree	Disagree
15. Everyone is capable of major crimes.	Agree	Disagree
16. Serious mental illness is best treated in hospital.	Agree	Disagree
17. More should be done for the mentally ill in the community.	Agree	Disagree
18. People must take responsibility for their actions.	Agree	Disagree
19. Generally, most people can be trusted.	Agree	Disagree
20. Everyone is bisexual to some degree.	Agree	Disagree

FIGURE 8.1 Beliefs and values questionnaire

Beliefs and Values Importance Questionnaire		
1. Most of my beliefs and values have stayed constant over the years.	Agree	Disagree
2. My beliefs and values are similar to those of my parents.	Agree	Disagree
3. I have changed many of my beliefs and values during the last 10 years.	Agree	Disagree
4. I can imagine changing many of them again in the next few years.	Agree	Disagree
5. There are certain core beliefs that I will never change.	Agree	Disagree
6. I have been influenced in my beliefs and values by one or two important people in my life.	Agree	Disagree
7. Religious beliefs play an important part in my life.	Agree	Disagree
8. I would like to be more clear about what I do and do not believe.	Agree	Disagree
9. It is important for me to be able to share my beliefs with other people.	Agree	Disagree
10. Most people have fixed beliefs once they reach a certain age.	Agree	Disagree

FIGURE 8.2 Beliefs and values importance questionnaire

REFLECTIONS

The idea of self-awareness has become a popular one in recent years. It is, however, problematic. If we consider the two words, we may be struck by the impossibility of the task in hand. If we are getting to know ourselves, 'what' is it that does the 'knowing'? We are asking that people reflect on themselves, who, in turn, are doing the reflecting. Perhaps this is a slightly academic point but it does raise the difficulty of getting to know oneself.

Perhaps the most straightforward way of considering self-awareness is the idea that we begin to get to know more about our thoughts, feelings and behaviour. More importantly, perhaps, we get to know more about how we relate to others and what they think about us. One model that helps, here, is the Johari window (Luft 1969). This consists of four domains as illustrated in Fig. 8.3. The main idea is that we come to know ourselves through two main means: self-disclosure and feedback from others. Thus, if we study the figure, we will see that if people know things about us and we know those things, the area is called the *open* area. If there are things that we know about ourselves but which are unknown to others, we have the *hidden* area. There

	Known to self	Not known to self
Known to others	Open area	Blind area
Not known to others	Hidden area	Unknown area

FIGURE 8.3 The Johari window

are also things that others know about us but of which we are unaware. This is the *blind* area. The people who devised the model speculate that there is a fourth area: that which is unknown to us and unknown to others. They call this the *unknown* area.

The authors further speculate that as we disclose information to others and as we get further feedback from others, so the various quadrants expand. Under conditions of *both* feedback from others and self-disclosure, they speculate that we get to know more about the unknown area.

It is interesting to 'play' with this model a little and to consider the degree to which *you* feel that it works. Consider the following questions:

■ What sorts of things do you know about yourself that are unknown to others?
■ What sorts of things do you share with some other people?
■ What sorts of things would you like other people to know about you and what would be the consequences?
■ What sorts of things do you speculate people think about you but do not disclose to you?
■ What would happen if people were really honest with you?
■ What would happen if you were really honest with others?
■ What stops you telling people how you *really* are?
■ What sort of people do you find it easy to disclose information to?
■ What do you find *most* difficult to disclose?
■ Is there anything that you have *never* disclosed to anyone?

Counselling is a disclosing activity. Sometimes, too, it involves the counsellor giving feedback to the client. It seems reasonable, then, for counsellors to have some experience of both self-disclosure and of feedback from others. Perhaps the counsellor should have a rather smaller 'unknown' area than other people. Perhaps, though, the unknown area is unbounded and, perhaps, as we get to know more about the unknown area, there is more to know.

Various arguments can be put forward for the development of self-awareness by nurses who counsel. First, there seems to be a relationship between the degree to which we can deal with our own emotional problems and those of others. If we have little insight into our own emotional difficulties, it seems likely that the problems of others are likely to 'throw us' when they occur. When we hear other people telling us about their problems and when we find that they are ones that resonate with our own (and we recognise that resonance for the first time), we are unlikely to be able to be therapeutic to the other person. While it is likely to be impossible to become totally self-aware, it seems reasonable to attempt to move a little way in this direction.

Another reason for becoming moderately self-aware is to make sure that we are clear of the boundaries between us and other people. Sometimes, when people talk about problems and difficulties, it is hard to differentiate between 'which problems are whose'. If we are self-aware and know something of our own problems, we are more likely to be able to keep a better sense of 'you out there and me in here' when relating to the client. Such boundaries are important. Again, if we merge our boundaries, we are less likely to be able to be therapeutic.

Finally, in this short list, self-awareness is useful in helping us to help ourselves. Counselling is hard work. We have problems, just as our clients have problems. Some degree of self-awareness is useful in helping us to work though our own difficulties. Sometimes, too, we can work through these with another person. Co-counselling offers one such framework for doing this.

Co-counselling

Co-counselling is a a process in which two people, who are trained in co-counselling, spend equal amounts of time in the roles of counsellor and client. Thus, for 1 hour, one of the pair works as client to the other's counsellor. After the hour, each person swaps roles. Training in co-counselling usually takes place thorough a 40-hour workshop either during the course of a week's workshop or on a part-time basis. Co-counselling is used for the following reasons:

- It is a means of developing listening skills.
- It can help to develop counselling interventions.
- It is a means of developing self-awareness.
- It can help to relieve stress.
- It can be used as a method of supervision.

Co-counsellors use certain conventions and techniques whilst working in the role of counsellor. The main quality and approach used is that of *listening* and *accepting*. The co-counsellor who is in the role of counsellor is never judgmental and always accepting. Thus, the process offers an ideal way of *modelling* these qualities for more 'formal' counselling relationships.

Second, co-counsellors never give advice. They limit themselves to the following sorts of interventions.

REFLECTION

This has been described in an earlier chapter. Reflection in co-counselling may consist of simply repeating a single word. An example of this sort of reflection is as follows:

'I felt uncomfortable when that happened.'
'Uncomfortable . . .'
'I was angry and I didn't know what to do. Although, in a way, I did know what to do.'

NOTING NON-VERBAL GESTURES

Here, the co-counsellor can either point to a gesture or indicate to the 'client' that he or she is gesticulating in a certain way and invite the 'client' to comment on it. Thus, the client is moving her arms in large circles and the counsellor asks 'What's happening with your arms? What are they 'saying'.

NOTING EMPHASES

Here, the counsellor reflects back emphasised words or phrases. An example of this is as follows:

'I started school and was *really* happy there.'
'You were *really* happy . . .'
'I was happier than I had ever been before. I have only just realised that!'

INVITING RECOLLECTION OF AN EARLY MEMORY

The counsellor notes that the client is talking about a potentially emotionally charged situation and invites the client to describe an early memory of this. An example is as follows:

'I was getting all worked up. Really upset. I didn't know what was going on in my life.'
'Can you remember the earliest time you felt like this?'
'When my father left home. When I was eight.'
'Can you describe that?'
'He just walked out. He left us all.'
'What are you feeling now?'
'Angry. Unhappy.'

And the pair explore those feelings.

USING AN EMPTY CHAIR

Here, the counsellor invites the client to imagine that someone that he or she is talking about is present, in the room. The counsellor then invites the client to have a 'conversation' with that person. This may sound like this:

'I always wanted to say that sort of thing to my mother, but never had the chance.'
'Imagine your mother is sitting in that chair. What do you want to say to her?'
'"I was happy when you were younger. It was easier then."'

'And what is she saying to you?'
'"It *was* easier then. We were all happier then. You have to make the best of it now/"'
'And what do you want to say to her?'
'"I can accept that. Thank you!"'
'What did that feel like?'
'It's sort of cleared the air. It feels different. I feel easier now.'

There is a range of other options open to the co-counsellor and details of these can be found elsewhere. The dialogue below offers an example of a co-counselling session.

Self-awareness questionnaire

As a further means of considering self-awareness, it it may be useful to be able to consider what areas of the self there are to consider. Sidney Jourard, the American psychologist, did a considerable amount of work on *self-disclosure*. He reviewed the condi-tions under which people disclosed themselves to others and came to the conclusion that *disclosure begets disclosure*. The person who readily discloses something of himself or herself to another person is also likely to invite disclosures from that other person. This does, of course, have implications for counselling, and raises the question of the degree to which nurses working as counsellors should be prepared to disclose themselves to clients. There are no hard and fast rules about this but some of the issues that should be borne in mind are as follows:

- Too much disclosure, too quickly, can frighten or put off some people.
- Too much disclosure shifts the balance of the relationship and the client may begin to feel that the counsellor has too many problems himself or herself to be counselling others.
- Disclosure may prematurely force another person into disclosing when that person is not ready.
- Self-disclosure by the counsellor may embarrass the client.

	Response
1. I am fairly happy with the way that I look.	
2. I think that I am reasonably popular with other people.	
3. There is at least one person to whom I can tell anything about myself.	
4. I have potential that is yet to be realised.	
5. I tend to underestimate myself.	
6. Compared with other people, I am fairly intelligent.	
7. Most people are more socially skilled than I am.	
8. I often have problems concentrating.	
9. I am best at doing things that I enjoy.	
10. I am fairly self-disciplined.	
11. I can be trusted with confidential information.	
12. I would like to be more physically attractive.	
13. I am confident about my sexuality.	
14. My live is generally going the way I want it to.	
15. I am prone to depressive moods.	
16. Most people are better than me.	
17. I am sensitive to the needs of others.	
18. I can be very selfish.	
19. I don't tolerate people I don't like very well.	

FIGURE 8.4 Self-awareness questionnaire

ACTIVITY BOX 8.2

The questionnaire shown in Fig. 8.4 offers you the chance to review some of the areas that are generally thought about under the heading 'self-awareness'. Consider each question and then think about the answers that you make to each of them. There are no right or wrong answers but answer the questions as honestly as you can. Be aware of any tendency that you have to exaggerate or simply to lie. Consider, too, using the questionnaire with another person. If you do this, you simply work through the questions and take it in turns to offer the answers to each item. In this way, you can do at least two things:

■ You can review your own levels of self-awareness.
■ You can satisfy some of the requirements of the Johari window by self-disclosing to another.

Definitions

Self-awareness is the process of gradually getting to know your thoughts, feelings and behaviours a little better. It is a lifelong process – one that is not particularly easy and one that has not been researched in any real detail. The general feeling seems to be that it is a good thing for those who counsel.

Co-counselling is a form of reciprocal counselling in which two people spend equal time each in the roles of counsellor and client. Each works as counsellor to the other and then both switch roles. It usually requires that the two people have attended a 40-hour training course. Such courses are often available at universities and extramural departments of universities and colleges.

DIALOGUE 8.1

The following dialogue is an example of two people engaging in 'one-side' of the co-counselling relationship. In this extract, the first person is acting as 'counsellor' to the other's 'client'.

'Let's make a start. Tell me what's happening for you at the moment.'
'I feel OK at the moment. Well, sort of.'
'Sort of . . .'
'Not very, actually. I'm angry, a bit. No, not angry, more agitated.'

'What's the agitation 'about'?'
'It's here, in the pit of my stomach.'
'When have you felt like this before? I mean, years ago, perhaps?'
'When I started at primary school.'
'Can you describe that?'
'I had to start school. I felt very young and very nervous. My mother was going to walk to school with me but she sort of fainted. I don't know what was wrong with her. Instead, my dad had to rush me to school before he went to work. I was very fond of him but I wanted my mother to be there on the first day and to sort of stay with me for a bit. Instead, my dad just dropped me off. And I had this feeling in my stomach, like it is now.'
'So what is the feeling *right now*?'
'It's changed. It's sort of bubbly and lighter. Excitement.'
'What are you excited about?'
'A relationship I'm having! It's good! I just realised, I sometimes confuse my feelings. Sometimes, I think it is *agitation* that I feel, when, instead, it's just excitement! That's helpful. I didn't realise that, before . . .'
'What's happening now?'
'I'm just taking that in. I'm thinking of how often I have done that in the past. And I'm thinking about how I don't *have* to do it. I could just accept that I get excited! Thanks!'

QUESTIONS ABOUT THE DIALOGUE

Read through the above co-counselling example and consider the following questions about it.

■ In what ways is the above dialogue similar to more 'formal' counselling?
■ In what ways is it different?
■ What does the *client* do that may not happen in more formal counselling?
■ What does the counsellor do that may not happen in more formal counselling?
■ Who 'holds the power' in the relationship?

REFLECTIONS

The session certainly follows a traditional pattern with the counsellor setting a clear starting point and asking the client how things are at the moment. The client then gives a clear indication that all is not well:

'I feel OK at the moment. Well, sort of.'

The counsellor remains client-centred and asks for some clarification about the term 'Sort of . . .'

The client then starts to explore feelings and admits to feeling agitated and, with the counsellor's focused questions, says that the locus of the agitation is the stomach.

The counsellor then takes a step that you would not normally find in 'formal' counselling by asking the client to identify when this feeling has happened before and places this in a time frame of 'years':

> 'When have you felt like this before? I mean, years ago, perhaps?'

It transpires that the client felt like this many years before in school, the first day at school, and that this was associated with being taken in by her father following the collapse of her mother. The counsellor does not explore this any further but brings the client right back to the present by asking:

> 'So what is the feeling *right now*?'

The client then gives a response that clearly changes the focus of the session by saying that the feeling has changed to one of excitement. Moving focus as quickly as this would not normally happen in 'formal' counselling because the counsellor would spend much more time exploring each facet in detail:

> 'It's changed. It's sort of bubbly and lighter. Excitement.'

The counsellor then brings the client into focus by asking:

> 'What are you excited about?'

The freedom associated with co-counselling has allowed the client to reach the conclusion that the excitement is related to a relationship that has just started and she realises that sometimes the adrenalin rush of excitement is sometimes confused with agitation. This is real enlightenment as the client had not realised this before:

> 'A relationship I'm having! It's good! I just realised, I sometimes confuse my feelings. Sometimes, I think it is *agitation* that I feel, when, instead, it's just excitement! That's helpful. I didn't realise that, before . . . '

The counsellor then asks the client to focus on the present and to share feelings; there is a real sense of liberation as the client realises that the shackles of what was perceived to be a negative feeling (agita-

tion) have been released and recognised as excitement:

> 'I'm just taking that in. I'm thinking of how often I have done that in the past. And I'm thinking about how I don't *have* to do it. I could just accept that I get excited! Thanks!'

The beauty of co-counselling is that it offers the opportunity for a relationship of equals. During this dialogue, the client had freedom to explore feelings at a rate that would not normally be acceptable in 'formal' counselling. This can be a liberating and enhancing process that can bring rewards and fulfilment for those involved.

ASSESSMENT ACTIVITY BOX

Read through this chapter and consider the following questions about yourself and about counselling.

- To what degreed to you consider yourself to be 'self-aware'?
- What else could you do to become more self-aware?
- What are your views about the notion of self-awareness?
- Do you feel that co-counselling might be useful to you?
- Do you know of training courses in co-counselling?
- If not, where would you go for that information?

Conclusion

This chapter has offered a brief introduction to the idea that self-awareness might be an important ingredient or personal quality in the nurse who wants to counsel. The idea that it can help in stress reduction and in the maintenance of boundaries between client and counsellor has been discussed. Co-counselling has been described as one means of developing self-awareness, and the Johari window has been identified as one means of conceptualising the concept of self-awareness.

9 COPING WITH PARTICULAR SITUATIONS

CHAPTER AIMS

- **To explore some potentially difficult situations**
- **To consider particular counselling situations in nursing**

Introduction

This chapter invites you to consider various counselling dialogues from nursing situations and asks you to think about how *you* would respond to them. All of them highlight either a potentially difficult ethical situation or one that is *practically* difficult. The former type of situation is one in which the rightness or wrongness of what is happening is in question. The latter type of situation is one in which it may be *difficult* to know how to respond. Before you read the dialogues, consider the following points that have to be addressed by anyone who works as a counsellor.

- The nature of counselling is such that people become fond of each other. More than that, the client may come to depend on the counsellor and/or vice versa. All counsellors need to consider strategies for dealing with this. One fairly common method of helping in these sorts of situations is *supervision*. Supervision is where another, more experienced counsellor meets with you to discuss, with you, your counselling.
- You may be attracted by the client or the client may be attracted by you. You need to think very carefully about whether or not it is in either of your interests to encourage this attraction – especially when it could lead to a deeper emotional or sexual relationship outside of the counselling relationship (this will build on the work you have already touched on in Chapter 3).
- Some problems in counselling are intractable –

there simply are not answers to everyone's problems. This limitation needs to be considered carefully and it is best to avoid glib reassurance.
- You may be faced with problems that you do not 'like'. You may have ethical or other objections to what the client is talking about. Again, you need to think carefully about whether or not you are the best person to help in this situation.

Bear in mind that there are no right or wrong ways of dealing with the situations occurring in the following dialogues. Each of them illustrates one of the issues described above. Discuss with a colleague the possible ways of dealing with each, and think about how *you* would work through the situations that have arisen. Consider, too, how you would have tried to *avoid* these situations arising.

DIALOGUE 9.1

'It's really good to be able to talk to you. No one really understands me in the way that you do.'

'I enjoy talking to *you*, you know. You shouldn't forget that.'

'Yes, but I often think about you when I'm at work and wonder what *you* would say about what I was doing. You seem to have some sort of almost magical way of knowing what I'm up to. I really appreciate that.'

'I couldn't do it if you weren't the person you are, you know. You're a very special person.'

DIALOGUE 9.2

'I'm not looking forward to going on holiday and not seeing you for nearly a month. What am I going to do then?'

'We'll have to face that when we get to it. I'm not sure what it will be like for me, not seeing you. These things work both ways.'

'We are both lucky, then, really.'

'I've looked forward to seeing you today.'

'Have you? What's that about, then? Do you like me?'

'Yes, of course I do.'

'I mean, really like me?'

'Yes, why do you ask?'

'Well, I think we are fairly close, don't you?'

'We are. Very close. I sometimes wonder if we aren't a bit too close. After all, I'm supposed to be your counsellor!'

'You're more than that, though.'

'You're more than one of my clients, too.'

'I sometimes wonder about seeing you outside of here.'

'We shouldn't, you know . . . '

'I'd like to . . . '

'A cup of coffee or a drink couldn't hurt, I suppose . . . '

DIALOGUE 9.3

'Things aren't much easier. My disability is making life impossible. The treatment for my illness is really making me ill and I can't seem to sort out my relationship with my wife. I think she doesn't really care for me any more but can't find a way of saying it.'

'I'm sure that the illness will improve. I mean, you're having the best treatment. And I'd be surprised if your wife really didn't love you.'

'She doesn't, you know. I know.'

'Of course you don't! That's just because of the side-effects of the medication you're on. Everyone feels like that.'

'Do they? Really? It's important, you know.'

'I know. And of course you will begin to feel better soon. Trust me.'

'I do. You know I do.'

'So, you have relationships with men as well as with women?'

'Yes. I have done for years now. The thing is, I'm really not sure whether or not I am really gay, or what.'

'But you've had successful relationships with women, haven't you?'

'Yes, I have. But I've also had good relationships with men, too?'

'Emotional ones, or just . . . sexual ones?'

'Both.'

'Is the emotional side of things more important to you?'

'I don't know.'

'And aren't you likely to have more satisfactory emotional relationships with women?'

'I don't see why? There are plenty of people who have relationships with other men . . . '

'But more people have longer lasting relationships with women, don't they?'

'Don't you like the idea that I might be gay?'

'It's not a question of what I think or what I don't think. It's what's best for you . . . '

QUESTIONS ABOUT THE DIALOGUES

When you have read the dialogues, ask yourself these questions:

- What did the counsellor do to help or hinder the development of the relationships?
- What are the 'rights and wrongs' of each?
- How might each situation have been handled better?
- What are your *personal* feelings about each situation?
- Have you ever been in a similar situation?
- If so, how did you deal with it?

REFLECTIONS DIALOGUE 9.1

Everyone enjoys being appreciated; it must be heartbreaking for people who give so much to a job but never feel as though anybody appreciates the effort they put in. Counselling people is no different, and knowing that you are appreciated by clients is a very rewarding part of the job. The first dialogue starts off with a really positive affirmation from the client:

'It's really good to be able to talk to you. No one really understands me in the way that you do.'

The counsellor warms to such ingratiating comments and responds in kind:

'I enjoy talking to *you*, you know. You shouldn't forget that.'

Then the conversation starts to develop in a way that should begin to ring warning bells for the counsellor:

> 'Yes, but I often think about you when I'm at work and wonder what *you* would say about what I was doing. You seem to have some sort of almost magical way of knowing what I'm up to. I really appreciate that.'

Rather than being client-centred, this sort of language seems to place the counsellor in a central position in the person's life. The most worrying point is the reference to the counsellor's 'magical way' of knowing what the client is up to. This is potentially very dangerous because the client is starting to view the counsellor as a sort of icon with pseudo-mystical powers. The counsellor needs to explore this with the client and dismiss any notion that what the client does outside of sessions can, in some way, be 'magically' tracked.

Instead of doing this, the counsellor seems to be captivated by the client's attentions and does nothing to address the wholly unrealistic position that has developed:

> 'I couldn't do it if you weren't the person you are, you know. You're a very special person.'

The problem with allowing this sort of problem to fester is that it is irreconcilable with any therapeutic theme. Receiving the adulation of clients must have its limits. Those limits come into most dangerous focus when it means that the client may have unrealistic expectations of the counselling relationship. If the client in this dialogue is talking about the counsellor having almost 'magical' insights, what mythical heights is counselling supposed to take both parties to? The real problem with this is that the counsellor is allowing the client to fantasise about the level of expectation that can be expected from the relationship. What should be concerned with getting the client to focus on issues has become a precarious scenario were the client embellishes the counsellor's ego – who will pick up the pieces when cold realisation dawns that the counsellor is only too human?

REFLECTIONS ON DIALOGUE 9.2

As we discussed in Chapter 3, being sexually attracted to another person is a key aspect of human nature. On a purely biological basis, if people were not attracted to each other the human species would, in time, become extinct. Society, however, has certain established conventions which provide a framework and avenue for the development of relationships. When a client comes to a counsellor, the foundation for their relationship has to be trust. Opening up and exploring issues that may have remained dormant for a long time means that the client is incredibly vulnerable.

In the second dialogue, the client expresses anxiety about a forthcoming holiday and not being able to see the counsellor:

> 'I'm not looking forward to going on holiday and not seeing you for nearly a month. What am I going to do then?'

The first part of the counsellor's response is perfectly acceptable:

> 'We'll have to face that when we get to it . . .'

However, the rest of the response is tarnished by moving attention from the client. In doing this, the counsellor creates the impression that the client will also be missed:

> 'I'm not sure what it will be like for me, not seeing you. These things work both ways.'

The client then takes the initiative that has been offered and infers that they are both fortunate to miss each other:

> 'We are both lucky, then, really.'

What follows is a frank exchange in which both parties talk about the affection they hold for each other. This is not a counselling session but two people gently exploring and divulging the way they feel about each other. The trouble is that the attraction has grown from a counselling relationship. This means that the client has shared very personal issues with the counsellor; this can lead to a position where that knowledge could be manipulated and abused.

The situation quickly tumbles towards an interpersonal relationship as the counsellor gives a brief and cursory mention about the counsellor–client relationship:

> 'We are. Very close. I sometimes wonder if we aren't a bit too close. After all, I'm supposed to be your counsellor!'

Within moments, the scene is set for their first date and the impartial, therapeutic basis of the counsellor–client relationship is gone for ever:

> 'I sometimes wonder about seeing you outside of here.'

'We shouldn't, you know . . .'
'I'd like to . . .'
'A cup of coffee or a drink couldn't hurt, I suppose . . .'

A key element of most training courses for counsellors is exploring the possibility of being sexually attracted to a client. In counselling, it occasionally happens that clients express their attraction for the counsellor. This is part and parcel of the therapeutic process; it seems natural that someone who may not have been attentively listened to before would find someone who offers total attention attractive. However, it is part of the counsellor's skill to fashion that attention into something positive that will, ultimately, improve the client's view of self and the world around them. Entering into an interpersonal relationship with a client confronts and destroys these ground rules.

REFLECTIONS ON DIALOGUE 9.3

Human sexuality is a very complex phenomenon that can be only partly explained by the labels we have for it. In the final dialogue, the client starts with a complex statement that has four important components:

1. His disability is making life impossible.
2. Treatment for his illness is making him ill.
3. He cannot sort out the relationship with his wife.
4. The client thinks that his wife no longer cares for him but cannot bring herself to say so.

Each of these points is vitally important and provides the counsellor with a menu of issues that all need to be carefully addressed. However, this counsellor deals with them in a quite dismissive manner by stating:

'I'm sure that the illness will improve. I mean, you're having the best treatment. And I'd be surprised if your wife really didn't love you.'

Such dismissiveness does not fudge the client as he insists that his wife no longer loves him; for some reason, the counsellor blames these perceptions on the medication:

'Of course you don't! That's just because of the side-effects of the medication you're on. Everyone feels like that.'

The emphasis then shifts to the client's sexuality, the man acknowledges a degree of confusion about his sexual preference:

'So, you have relationships with men as well as women.'
'Yes. I have done for years now. The thing is, I'm really not sure whether or not I am really gay, or what.'

The counsellor then tries to establish whether or not the relationship the client has with other men is emotional or sexual (note the emphasis on *just sexual*, as if sexual fulfilment was much less important than the emotional sort):

'Emotional ones, or just . . . sexual ones?'

It is difficult to see the counsellor's point here – how can emotion be divorced from the sexual and vice versa? Compartmentalising feelings in this way is a limited way to view the human condition.

The final straw comes for the client when the counsellor argues that the majority of men have longer relationships with women; this provokes the client to charge the counsellor with the following question:

'Don't you like the idea that I might be gay?'

The counsellor, after asking a series of questions that reflect personal values, then retreats behind the counselling 'nutmeg' that focus should remain with the client by saying:

'It's not a question of what I think or what I don't think. It's what's best for you . . .'

This dialogue reveals some very poor work by the counsellor. The questions and comments mask a 'hidden agenda' that suggests the client's sexuality is causing a problem. When a client confronts a counsellor with the open charge of 'Don't you like the idea that I might be gay?', then the session has gone horribly wrong and means that the counsellor has transferred prejudice; such themes have no place in a therapeutic relationship that is supposed to be based on trust and honesty.

ASSESSMENT ACTIVITY BOX

Review the chapter and begin to formulate the questions that you need to ask *yourself* about various aspects of counselling. Consider, in particular, the following issues:

■ How much and what sort of training should you have?

ASSESSMENT ACTIVITY BOX – *(contd)*

- Do you have facilities for being supervised if you counsel?
- How do you deal with interpersonal stress?
- How do you cope with ambiguity?
- Is counselling something that you really want to do?
- To what degree are you already counselling?
- What do you need to do next, professionally and personally?

Conclusion

This chapter has considered some of the sorts of ethical and practical problems that can arise in everyday counselling in nursing and other situations. The temptation to develop co-dependence is a strong and very human one. However, if both the client and the counsellor are to thrive in the relationship, this issue must be met head on. Also, it is essential that anyone doing counselling knows their limits. Finally, our own prejudices and preferences are bound to show through in what we do as counsellors and nurses. We need, then, constantly to review our own performance and our own systems of beliefs and values.

10 COUNSELLING AND PALLIATIVE CARE

Introduction

You may ask why we have devoted a whole chapter to the issue of counselling and palliative care? In answer, it can be said that counselling of this sort is quite unique, simply because you often only have one chance to get it right as people only die once. Other forms of counselling can often be redeemed when mistakes have been made – such opportunities are rare when counselling the dying; work of this sort really is akin to walking in a moral minefield and makes tremendous demands on the counselling skills of nurses.

We are all going to die. In a world of few certainties, the absolute nature of human mortality remains constant. Fear of death, or perhaps, more fundamentally, what the process of dying will involve, is both common and primal to us all. To a large extent, this reflects a biological instinct to survive; it is needed for the continuation of the human species. This theme is further compounded by a societal trend to treat all things relating to death and dying as taboo. With a focused piece of writing, May (1969: 106) offers a penetrative and powerful reflection which is steeped with the sort of language that explains why talk of death and dying is frowned upon in most parts of the social milieu:

> Death is obscene, unmentionable, porno-graphic ... death is a nasty mistake. Death is not to be talked of in front of the children, nor talked about at all if we can help it.

Those of us who have direct contact with dying patients may find it difficult to identify with May's evocative demand that talk of death be avoided. Nursing, as a profession, has always viewed honesty as an important virtue and has placed it high on the moral agenda. This has been reinforced and propagated by the stereotypical myth of the nurse as an 'angel' (Holloway 1992). Such an image is supported by an almost gut reaction against the possibility that a nurse could ever justifiably tell a lie. Yet dilemmas of practice do cast down challenges to the notion that truth can always be upheld as a universal virtue. Reflecting this theme, Kendrick and Kinsella (1994: 215) state 'The truth is often hidden behind a veil of secrecy and mystique – lifting it can create both light and shadow'.

Oscar Wilde, the Victorian playwright, author and poet, once remarked, with typical whimsical insight, that 'the truth is rarely pure, and never simple'. Such wisdom certainly portrays the difficulties involved with counselling patients who are dying and their loved ones.

Counselling and risk

A great deal of this chapter is concerned with risk. Each time you decide to engage with another human being, you metaphorically 'roll a dice'. You can never know, before an event, how it will turn out. Just a simple reflection on some of your own personal encounters should show the unpredictable nature of human dynamics. By this stage in the book, we hope that the issues explored have graphically illustrated some of the complexities that can emerge in both counselling and caring.

A nurse should always seek to avoid harming a patient; however, all interventions carry a degree of risk, which may result in harm being caused. Every human activity carries with it degree of risk. Commenting on the relationship between all actions and risk, Stewart (1992: 329) states:

> The degree of risk is the extent to which harm may result from a particular action. There are many different kinds of risk, including economic risk, the risk to life and health and the risk to the environment. Risk is not the same as danger. Walking downstairs carries a definite degree of risk: it is one of the commonest causes of accidents in the home. But you

would hardly call it dangerous. In our daily lives we all risk being involved in accidents. If you ride in a car, it may crash. If you choose to walk, a car may hit you. If you stay at home and light the gas, the house may catch fire.

Problems start to arise when patients do not feel that the harm caused by an intervention can be justified by the net outcome. Taking this further, a person may feel that to suffer the consequences of chemotherapy – alopecia, diarrhoea, depression and skin soreness – could not justify a short remission from cancer.

What this highlights is that it is not sufficient to think of ethics purely in terms of doing good and avoiding harm. The main point is to avoid acting dangerously and trying to ensure that the end result of an action justifies any harm caused. To illustrate this, if a patient, who is paralysed down the left side, slips when being helped out of the bath by two nurses following hospital policy about lifting and handling, then it is probably an accident; however, if the patient slips because a nurse is trying to do the lift single-handed, then it is probably an example of dangerous practice. Thus, a degree of risk is acceptable; it can never be wholly eliminated but efforts should always be made to keep the chances of harm occurring to a minimum.

Estimating risk and doing everything possible to avoid harm is an important part of using counselling skills. When one of the authors (K.K.) was a final-year student nurse, a 68-year-old man with advanced lung cancer – we'll call him 'David' – asked if he could have 'a word'. The conversation went something like this (David was a retired Enrolled Nurse):

DIALOGUE 10.1

'It's been 5 days since I've had that biopsy done yet nobody's been in to give me the results. I'm fed up having scans and investigations – I just want to know the truth.'

'Have any of the doctors had a word with you about the results?'

'Everytime I ask the doctors for some honest answers they keep telling me they're waiting for results – I know I've had enough tests done to find out what's wrong with me.'

'If it's OK with the charge nurse, would you like me to tell you the results of the tests?'

'Yeh, I just want someone to confirm what I already know.'

At this point, I (K.K.) left and asked the charge nurse if it was OK for me to tell David that he was not going to get better. The charge nurse said that if I felt confident enough to deal with the situation, I could tell David about the test results. The rest of the conversation went something like this:

'David, there's never any easy way to give news like this but . . .'

'It's OK lad, you can stop right there – just tell me one thing, has it spread everywhere?'

'Yes, Dave, the scan shows it's spread everywhere.'

'Thanks for telling me "how it is" – just give me a bit of time by myself would you.'

'I'm really sorry David – just ring the bell if there's anything you want. I'll come back and see you later anyway.'

ACTIVITY BOX 10.1

- Read the above dialogue again.
- What would you have said to David when he said: 'Thanks for telling me "how it is" – just give me a bit of time by myself would you'.

REFLECTIONS

An hour later, I (K.K.) knocked on the door of David's room. There was no answer. Pensively, I slowly opened the door – the first thing I saw was blood running down the opposite wall. On the bed, David lay motionless in a massive pool of blood – it seemed to cover the whole room. He had cut his carotid artery.

David had decided to take his own life rather than be ravaged by terminal cancer. In a way, it could be viewed as an act of proclamation – deciding to take his life before life took his dignity, freedom and individuality. When using counselling skills with David, I had taken a risk; it was his choice to die, having been given the truth about his condition. However, for a long time after, it made me (K.K.) question whether or not patients should be told the truth about a terminal prognosis.

No matter how experienced we become, the question 'Am I going to die, nurse?' never becomes easy to answer. There is nothing vague or ambiguous about the question. We do not have to use mirroring skills or explore the cues to make further inferences; the question is simply put and very direct. Indeed, it is this focused approach that can catch us off guard. There is nowhere to hide when a dying person makes such an enquiry and the choice is clear – we either lie or tell the truth.

There are usually two main reasons that are put forward to support lying:

1. Adherence to the principle 'do no harm'.
2. Patients do not want to know the truth.

As we have already seen, the notion that health care delivery can ever be 'free of harm' is utopian. If a person has the courage to ask so plainly about their mortality, then he or she deserves to be answered in a similar fashion. This does not mean that revealing the truth to a person about their impending death will be easy – for either the patient or the nurse – but it does free the dying person to face death with an open and informed gaze.

In relation to the second premise in defence of lying, there is little doubt that some patients do not want to be told the truth about their impending mortality. However, Bok (1978) revealed that 80 per cent of patients wanted to know the truth about their condition and prognosis. Supporting this approach, Gillon (1986: 105) states 'There are difficulties to overcome, but avoiding deceit is a basic moral norm, defensible from several moral perspectives'. Similar themes are echoed by Faulder (1985: 89) who states 'In asking patients to trust them it would seem only fair that doctors should reward that trust by dealing honestly with them'. All of this must be tempered by the notion that news of a poor diagnosis should always be revealed as gently as possible and in a way that is dictated by the patient.

The consequences of not dealing truthfully with a dying person can be catastrophic. Sometimes, practitioners enter into the fragile world of word games to try and avoid a direct confrontation with the truth. Over the years, we have heard many vague and evasive responses to the question 'Am I going to die, nurse?'; for example:

'We are all going to die, the big question is when'.
'I thought the doctor told you that it was a tumour – I never heard the word cancer mentioned.'
'What sort of a question is that to ask when you are looking so well?'

Nurses sometimes hide behind such words, phrases and empty semantics when faced with difficult questions. A host of popular terms are used to try

and validate lies or deception. Challenging such themes, we do not 'disguise the truth', 'tell fibs' or offer 'white lies'. Such terms are mere rhetoric – we either lie or tell the truth. Terms such as 'to be economical with the truth' are a moral smoke screen.

If we do decide to keep the truth of impending death from a patient, then it can violate any of the therapeutic themes which have been established. To be the victim of lies and deceit at the end of one's life can volley the dying person into a disenfranchised state where those who were thought to be trustworthy become the conduits of subterfuge.

The only substantial reason that would justify a dying person being left in a state of unknowing is a clear expression, from them, of not wanting to hear about a terminal prognosis. To impose such news on someone who did not want to know it confronts autonomy and trust in much the same way as withholding such information does to the individual who expresses a desire to know. Surely, such themes can never be compatible with the resonance of counselling as a therapeutic tool.

This section has explored some of the difficult moral themes that surround counselling a patient who asks 'Am I going to die, nurse?' An equally difficult scenario surrounds the troubling issue of collusion. This is the delicate scenario that involves relatives or loved ones demanding that the truth of a dire prognosis be kept from the patient. Commenting on the precarious nature of such themes, Ballinger (1997: 44) comments:

Using deception in health care is a high risk strategy. Truth telling is a basic moral principle for health workers to abide by. The decision for non-disclosure of the truth or to withhold vital information concerning the patient can have important effects on the doctor–patient and nurse–patient relationships and can impinge on the patient's rights to information.

Collusion, counselling and the moral maze

It may be said, with reasonable certainty, that truth and honesty are central themes in relationships between patients and practitioners. In most cases, to deal in anything other than the truth can violate trust and destroy any hope of a therapeutic association; the key problem with collusion is that it confronts these themes from the misplaced notion that it offers protection.

ACTIVITY BOX 10.2

Consider the following scenario based on a real event from practice; all names used are fictitious.

John is 14 years old and has been suffering with early-morning nausea and vomiting, violent headaches and an inability to concentrate on his school work. The GP thought that this was a virus which would pass in a week or two. However, the symptoms progressively got worse and included faints and a feeling of numbness down the left-hand side of his body. John was immediately referred to the regional neurological centre for investigations.

The result of these investigations was devastating. John was found to have a particularly aggressive, malignant tumour. Unfortunately, the growth was fixed to vital structures, which meant that surgery was not a viable option. John's parents, Jane and Michael, were extremely upset by this news. The consultant neurologist was gently honest and said that the most that could be done was to make John as comfortable as possible in the time that was left to him. Jane and Michael were enraged; why could nothing be done for their son? – 'There must be something you can do – he's only fourteen'. The dreadful reality was that nothing could be offered to John and his parents except the fervent hope and desire that palliative care could keep him pain free and comfortable.

Five days after hearing the news of John's prognosis, Jane and Michael ask to see the senior sister, Pauline Houlton. Looking drawn and exhausted, Jane starts to plead with Pauline, 'Sister, Mike and I have had a chance to think things through about John. It's really nice that you feel able to say his illness will be closely watched and everything done to make him comfortable – that reassures us – but something else is really bothering us'.

Jane starts to cry and Pauline sits quietly waiting for her to carry on in her own time, Mike interjects, 'The point is that we don't want John to know about his illness. At the moment he still thinks that he has a virus. He really couldn't take the news that there was nothing more that could be done ... so if he asks what is wrong he mustn't be told the truth – he just could not take it, for goodness sake, he's our little boy'.

Jane and Mike cling to each other, both weeping bitterly. Pauline leaves them, at what she feels is an intensely private moment, and ponders the dilemma which the team now face.

Questions

- Should Pauline agree with Mike's and Jane's request?
- What would you do if placed in Pauline's position?

REFLECTIONS

The type of dilemma that Pauline is being asked to engage in is typical of the complex web woven by people involved with collusion. It involves an understanding that the news of a poor prognosis be kept from the patient. The mores that inform interaction between people would not normally tolerate this form of dynamic. However, such views are confronted when relatives or significant others put forward the sort of powerful sentiments that have occurred in the previous scenario. Relatives who seek collusion often argue that they are in a much better position to understand what their loved one can and cannot take.

Reflecting upon the reasons why relatives put forward requests such that the truth of a poor prognosis be kept from the patient, Kendrick and Shea (1995: 9) comment:

A prognosis which indicates that death is inevitable confronts the most primal elements of the human condition. It is understandable that relatives sometimes request or even demand that such devastatingly 'bad news' be kept from a loved one. The essential reason for this is to try and protect the dying person from the ravages inherent to such an announcement. Underpinning this is a firm belief that it is in the dying person's 'best interests' not to know that death is approaching.

What emerges from this is a convincing mandate from John's parents to keep the truth from him. Initially, this can take both a direct and an indirect form. If John was to specifically ask what was wrong with him, then the nurse being questioned could either omit to tell the truth by, for example, conveniently 'sidestepping' the issue – a common ruse being 'I'll get the doctor to have a word with you'. Alternatively, the nurse may choose to take the more direct route and lie to John by saying, for example, 'These viruses can take an eternity to clear up'. Approaches of this nature are usually offered under the guise of a patriarchal impulse that is intended to protect the patient from the truth. Despite the good intent that may support such themes, a host of ethical indicators highlight the harm that can emerge from such reasoning.

The destruction of truth

The very nature of collusion means that truth will be a casualty. If practitioners and relatives enter into a covert understanding which alienates a dying person from knowledge of the prognosis, then the threads of a therapeutic bond become violated and torn. What can emerge from this is a scenario born of deceit and disingenuous encounters. The intent underpinning collusion is often to protect the dying person from the news of an inevitable death from a pathology that cannot be cured. Unfortunately, once such a position is taken, it can have dire repercussions for the dynamics between all those involved with the dying person. Reflecting on these themes, Kendrick and Kinsella (1994: 212) state:

> Once we have entered into the dangerous scenario of collusion it leads to a constant striving to avoid tumbling down the slippery slope into a swirling vortex of lies, misrepresentation and fabrication.

Returning once more to the earlier scenario, Jane and Mike would love to protect John from the news of the brain tumour and what it will inevitably mean. However, the loss of autonomy and trust which can result from collusion can hardly be justified – the opportunity for John to reflect on his life and make sense of it should be not be stolen from him under the guise of beneficence. In a seminal work on medical ethics, the moral theologian Bernard Haring (1974: 45) explores the ethical issues surrounding collusion and states:

> Loving care for the dying is one of the supreme expressions of our respect for the human person and of truthful relationship with him ... To deceive a dying person about the most crucial personal and awesome fact of his life, his approaching death, is to treat him like an object. It can mean robbing him of the most decisive act of freedom.

The use of the word 'object' gives the thrust of Haring's argument definite focus and direction. What this establishes is that in colluding against the truth, relatives and practitioners deny the dying person the status of being a valued subject. In logical sequence, this inevitably means that the patient becomes an object. This shift in perception and emphasis has a long history in the way that dying people are treated (Menzies 1970, McIntosh 1977, Hanson 1994). The cliché which is often used to highlight this shift from valued subject to object is when a practitioner refers to the patient as, for example, 'the CA in the side ward'.

This part of the chapter has dealt with the difficult ethical themes involved with collusion. We have discovered that the beneficent base that is used to support collusion crumbles when faced with the affront it can cause to honesty, openness, autonomy and trust. Commenting upon the destructive aspects of deceit, Korsgaard (1986) cites Immanuel Kant, who stated 'Whatever militates against frankness lowers the dignity of man'. Practitioners sometimes use language as a veil to hide from their own vulnerability and fear of mortality. This flailing in the shadows of semantics is understandable, but denying someone access to the truth about the nature of a terminal illness not only shatters any basis for an open dialogue but threatens the therapeutic themes which palliative care can offer.

Conclusion

The key task of this chapter has been to examine counselling in relation to palliative care and truth telling. Revealing to patients and their loved ones that death is fast approaching may evoke feelings of horror and disbelief. However, there may also be a feeling of relief – that at least something has been found which can be labelled and seen as the cause of illness. Professional experience often reveals that patients find the 'not knowing' more unbearable than the harsh reality that life is coming to an end (Hanson 1994). Being honest about a prognosis which indicates that life will end does give the patient a tremendous blow. However, such news, if offered gently and with a velvet glove, is easier to take than the devastation of trust and honesty which lying and deceit would mean for the dying person.

It is extremely difficult to envisage a situation in palliative care where lying could ever be morally justified. We have argued that the therapeutic relationship between the nurse and a dying person becomes shallow, defiled and even irreconcilable once lying and deceit have entered. The patient's vulnerability adds another dimension to the importance of truthfulness – to lie to such a person hacks at the structures on which so many frail defences are placed. To expose patients to such an affront can rarely be justified within a process so intrinsically concerned with caring. The alternative to honesty and openness is a scenario of hushed whispers, hidden agendas, collusion, deceit and lying – surely, such elements can never be reconcilable with the central themes of nursing, counselling and caring (Kendrick and Weir 1996).

11 A DEBATE ABOUT COUNSELLING

The preceding chapters have all been about various aspects of the counselling process. Also in those chapters, we have outlined some of the ethical principles that need to be considered in counselling. In this final chapter, a variety of issues are raised about counselling as a whole. The point of this debate is not to answer questions but to encourage you to debate the points, both with yourself and with others.

Is counselling a 'special' process?

First, is counselling different to simply 'talking to' people? After all, we all have conversations with our families and friends and sort things out in an informal way. Can we say, then, that what counsellors do is markedly different to what we all do when we have conversations with people we know? If it *is* the same as ordinary conversation, then we might not need to have special training to do it – for, as we have established, most of us are already quite skilled in talking to other people. If it is *not* the same as ordinary conversation, we would be bound to say in *what ways* it is different. We might say, for example, that counsellors *listen* more carefully. This would seem a reasonable claim but the counter-claim might be made that *lots of people* listen well. If they do not, we might train them simply to improve their listening skills.

We might say that counsellors have 'special insights' into other people's problems. But this has been largely ruled out, by Carl Rogers' claim that it is the *client* who is the expert on his or her own problems. If this *is* the case, then it may be the client who is the expert and not the counsellor – at least when it comes to 'special insights'. What Rogers seems to be claiming is that each person has his or her own special insights and that what the counsellor does is to help that person to find them.

Any claims that counsellors have 'special knowl-

edge' or 'psychological insights' that other people do not have are bound to be debatable. It would suggest, perhaps, that counsellors are in some way able to stand outside of the 'general' human condition and to commentate on it or study it in some way. This seems an unlikely state of affairs.

We are left, then, with the debate about *exactly* what counselling is that distinguishes it from other sorts of conversations. As we have seen, right at the start of this book, people have tried to separate it out from its partner, psychotherapy, and we have noted, too, that some have argued that it is almost *impossible* to do this. And yet if counselling is to survive, it seems likely to be necessary, at some point, to be able to define, with some precision, exactly what counselling is.

Are people the experts on their own problems?

We have noted, at various points in this text, that, as a rule, counsellors take the view that it is the individual who has the key to his or her own problems. The argument goes something like this. I live a different life to you, I have a different history, I have different experiences, beliefs and values and I have a certain 'uniqueness'. All of these things contribute to the notion that only I can decide for myself. You cannot decide for me. This is, of course, *strictly* true: you cannot *make* me decide anything. In the end, I have to decide things for myself. What is less clear, though, is the degree to which you might or might not attempt to *influence* me in my decision making. Carl Rogers seemed fairly clear on this point: it is best *not* to try. However, other points of view are possible.

First, we might question the degree to which we really do differ as people. Rather than stress our individuality, we might note our *similarities*. In many ways, people are more similar to each other than they are different. If this is the case (and you may disagree), then it seems reasonable to suggest that two people *may* attempt to influence each other in their decision-making processes. After all, in 'ordinary' conversations about problems, with family and friends, we do tend to do this.

Second, many people have hard-won experience. If you have lived a reasonable length of time, it is likely that you have had a range of life experiences. It might be argued that it is a shame, sometimes, *not* to share these experiences with another person as a means of helping them to think through their decision making. Sharing experiences in this way does nothing to alter the fact that, in the end, *I* have to make up my *own* mind about what I do and what I do not do. I can either listen to your experiences and decide that some of the things you have experienced are useful for me, or I can choose to reject your experiences. However, if I have not *heard* those experiences, I have no such choice.

Are people 'essentially good'?

This is a particularly thorny issue. Carl Rogers' writings seem to suggest that he felt that people were basically good. This, as we have discussed, is not a new idea; nor is the idea that people are 'essentially bad'. Another point of view, however, is that 'good' and 'bad' are social constructs – notions developed over time, by societies in which people live. Thus, it is society at any given time that determines whether or not an action is good or bad. A simple example will suffice here. In wartime, killing certain people is deemed good (or at least acceptable). In peacetime, killing people is deemed bad (except in certain societies in which it is viewed as being the appropriate approach to dealing with other people who have killed someone). The idea that 'killing is bad' is, at least to some degree, debatable and variable. Goodness and badness, then, may depend on time, context, society, situation, and so on. The idea that we are all *born* good or bad is a tricky one, but one that is linked, inextricably, with many theological positions.

The other point that may be made here is that if we are to argue that people are *essentially* good,

does this mean that they are always capable of being helped to be good? Or, are there circumstances in which the goodness 'goes wrong'? If so, what are those circumstances and how might they be dealt with? Furthermore, is *everyone* essentially good or are there people born who are exceptions? The same sorts of points may be made about essential 'badness'. If people are essentially bad, can they be made good and in what circumstances?

What are the limits of accepting clients?

In Carl Rogers' writings there is a considerable emphasis on the need for the counsellor to accept the client – in almost all respects. We should accept what he or she says and we should accept that these are the 'true' feelings of that client. The suggestion, then, is that we do not disagree with, argue with or reject what the client says. It is worth considering to what degree we can *always* accept what another person says to us. Might we, for example, accept, fully, the fact that someone is telling us that he wants to kill himself? Does accepting, in this situation, mean *agreeing* that the person is free to kill himself? Or, should we accept that the client wants to kill himself but prevent him from doing so? If we do this, are we still 'accepting' the client in every respect?

If a client tells us that he is abusing another person, is what he tells us 'acceptable' or should we seek to encourage him to stop? If we encourage him away from abusive behaviour, are we in some ways not accepting him completely?

Clearly, in both of the above situations it would seem that common sense tells us that intervention of some sort is required. In most situations, faced with a person who is telling us that they are going to kill themselves, we would be tempted to try to ensure that they do not. In most situations in which a person is abusing another person, we are likely to want to discourage them from doing so. The question remains: to what degree is such intervention going against the 'acceptance' rule? And, once this rule is breached, how many sorts of exceptions can we make to the rule? Indeed, is it a 'rule' at all? Or, would we be safer in saying something like 'where possible, it is valuable to accept the other person'?

REFERENCES

Abrams, N.A. 1978: A contrary view of the nurse as patient advocate. *Nursing Forum* **17**(1), 260–6.

Adshead, G. and Dickenson, D. 1993: Why do doctors and nurses disagree? In Dickenson, D. and Johnson, M. (eds), *Death, Dying and Bereavement*. Sage, London, 161–8.

Allmark, P. and Klarzynski, R. 1992: The case against nurse advocacy. *British Journal of Nursing* **2**(1), 33–7.

Aptekar, H.H. 1955: *The Dynamics of Casework and Counselling*. Houghton Mifflin, Cambridge, MA.

Assay, J.L. and Herbert, J.M. 1983: Who is the seductive patient? *American Journal of Nursing*, April, 530–2.

Ballinger, D. 1997: Is it ever acceptable to deceive a patient? *Nursing Times* **27**(93), 44–5.

Bok, S. 1978: *Lying: Moral Choice in Public and Private Life*. Pantheon, New York.

Breese, J. 1983: Counselling pupils in centres for disruptives. *Maladjustment and Therapeutic Education* **1**(1), 6–12.

British Association for Counselling (BAC) 1989: *Code of Ethics and Practice for Counselling Skills*. BAC, Rugby.

Brown, J.M., Kitson, A. and McKnight, T.J. 1992: *Challenges in Caring: Explorations in Nursing and Ethics*. Chapman & Hall, London.

Brown, M. 1985: Matter of commitment. *Nursing Times* **81**(18), 26–7.

Buber, M. 1958: *I and Thou*. Scribner, New York.

Burnard, P. 1994: *Counselling Skills for Health Professionals*, 2nd edn. Chapman & Hall, London.

Campbell, A.V. 1984a: *Moderated Love*. SPCK, London.

Chadwick, R.F. and Tadd, W. 1992: *Ethics and Nursing Practice: A Case Study Approach*. Macmillan Press, Basingstoke.

Cinebell, H.J. 1966: *Basic Types of Pastoral Counselling*. Abingdon Press, New York.

Concise Oxford Dictionary, The 1992: Oxford University Press, Oxford.

Crompton, M. 1992: *Children and Counselling*. Edward Arnold, London.

Curtin, L. and Flaherty, M.J. 1982: *Nursing Ethics: Theories and Pragmatics*. Prentice-Hall, Englewood Cliffs, NJ.

Dalrymple, T. 1996: Seen a happy counsellor? *The Sunday Times*, 7th January.

Dickson, D.A., Hargie, O. and Morrow, N.C. 1989: *Communication Skills Training for Health Professionals: An Instructor's Handbook*. Chapman & Hall, London.

Dryden, W., Charles-Edwards, D. and Woolfe, R. 1989: *Handbook of Counselling in Britain*. Tavistock/Routledge, London.

Egan, G. 1986: *Exercises in Helping Skills*, 3rd edn. Brooks/Cole, Monterey, CA.

Faulder, C. 1985: *Whose Body is It?: The Troubling Issue of Informed Consent*. Virago, London.

French, P. 1993: *Social Skills for Nursing Practice*, 2nd edn. Chapman & Hall, London.

French, W.L. and Raven, C.A. 1959: *The Basis of Social Power*. University of Michigan Press, East Lansing, MI.

Frost, M. 1974: *Nursing Care of the Schizophrenic Patient*. Kimpton, London.

Garmarnikow, E. 1978: The sexual division of labour: the case of nursing. In Kuhn, A. and Wolpe, P. (eds), *Feminism and Materialism: Women and Modes of Production*. Routledge & Kegan Paul, London, 218–36.

Gillon, R. 1986: *Philosophical Medical Ethics*. Wiley, Chichester.

Hanson, E. 1994: *The Cancer Nurse's Perspective*. Quay, Lancaster.

Hargie, O., Saunders, C. and Dickson, D. 1981: *Social Skills in Interpersonal Communication*, 2nd edn. Croom Helm, London.

Haring, B. 1974: *Medical Ethics*. St Paul Publications, Slough.

Henry, C. and Pashley, G. 1990: *Health Ethics*. Quay, Lancaster.

Holloway, J. 1992: Media representations of the nurse. In Soothill, K., Henry, I.C. and Kendrick, K. (eds), *Themes and Perspectives in Nursing*. Chapman & Hall, London, 16–40.

Holmes, J. and Lindley, R. 1991: *The Values of Psychotherapy*. Oxford University Press, Oxford.

Hopson, B. 1981: Counselling and healing. In Griffiths, D. (ed.), *Psychology and Medicine*. Macmillan, London.

Janis, I.L,, Houland, P. and Kelly, H. 1959: *Personality and Persuadability*. Yale University Press, New Haven, CT.

Jones, A. 1994: *Counselling Adolescents: School and After*. Kogan Page, London.

Kendrick, K.D. 1991: Partners in passing: ethical aspects of nursing the dying person. *International Journal of Advances in Health and Nursing Care* **1**(1), 11–27.

Kendrick, K. 1994: An advocate for whom – doctor or patient? How far can a nurse be a patient's advocate? *Professional Nurse* **9**(12), 826–9.

Kendrick, K. 1995a: Ethical pathways in cancer and palliative care. In David, J. (ed.), *Cancer Care: Prevention, Treatment and Palliation*. Chapman & Hall, London, 224–44.

Kendrick, K. 1995b: Nurses and doctors: a problem of partnership. In Soothill, K., Mackay, L. and Webb, C. (eds), *Interprofessional Relations in Health Care*. Edward Arnold, London, 239–52.

Kendrick, K.D. 1995c: Accountability and interprofessional relationships. *Professional Nurse* (in conjunction with Thames Valley University) **10**(9) (card insert).

Kendrick, K.D. 1997: What is advancing nursing practice. *Professional Nurse* **12**(10), 689.

Kendrick, K.D. and Kinsella, M. 1994: 'Lifting the veil': truth-telling in palliative care. *International Journal of Cancer Care* **3**(4), 211–15.

Kendrick, K. and Shea, T. 1995: With velvet gloves: the ethics of collusion. *Palliative Care Today* **IV**(1), 8–11.

Kendrick, K. and Weir, P. 1996: Truth telling in palliative care: a nursing response. In Soothill, K., Henry, I.C. and Kendrick, K. (eds), *Themes and Perspectives in Nursing*, 2nd edn. Chapman & Hall, London, 218–29.

Kitson, A.L. 1991: *Therapeutic Nursing and the Hospitalised Elderly*. Scutari Press, Harrow, 23, 220.

Korsgaard, C.M. 1986: The right to lie. Kant on dealing with evil. *Philosophy and Public Affairs* **15**(336), 133–56.

Lawrence, Brother 1981: *The Practice of the Presence of God*. Hodder & Stoughton, Sevenoaks.

Lawler, J. 1991: *Behind the Screens: Nursing, Somology and the Problem of the Body*. Churchill Livingstone, Edinburgh.

Lewin, E. 1977: Feminist ideology and the meaning of work: the case of nursing. *Catalyst* **10**(11), 90–8.

Ley, P. 1982: Satisfaction, compliance and communication. *British Journal of Clinical Psychology* **21**, 241–54.

Luft, J. 1969: *Of Human Interaction*. Mayfield, Palo Alto, CA.

Mackay, L. 1989: *Nursing a Problem*. Open University Press, Milton Keynes.

Mackay, L. 1993: *Conflicts in Care. Medicine and Nursing*. Chapman & Hall, London

Mallon, B. 1987: *An Introduction to Counselling Skills for Special Educational Needs*. Manchester University Press, Manchester.

May, R. 1969: *Love and Will*. Dell, New York.

McIntosh, I. 1977: *Communication and Awareness in a Cancer Ward*. Croom Helm, London.

Menzies, I. 1970: *Communication and Stress: A Nursing Perspective*. Macmillan, London.

Murphy, C. and Hunter, C. 1984: *Ethical Problems in the Nurse–Patient Relationship*. Allyn & Bacon, Boston, MA.

Nelson-Jones, R.. 1995: *The Theory and Practice of Counselling*, 2nd edn. Cassell, London.

Noonan, E. 1983: *Counselling Young People*. Methuen, London.

Parnell, J.W. and Kendrick, K. 1995: *Study Skills for Nurses: A Practical Guide*. Churchill Livingstone, Edinburgh.

Pearson, A. and Vaughan, B. 1986: *Nursing Models for Practice*. Heinemann, London.

Penn, K. 1994: Patient advocacy in palliative care. *British Journal of Nursing* **3**(1), 40–2.

Penner, L. 1978: *Social Psychology: A Contemporary Approach*. Oxford University Press, Oxford.

Reber, A. 1985: *The Penguin Dictionary of Psychology*. Penguin, Harmondsworth.

Reyner, J.H. 1984: *the Gurdjieff Inheritance*. Turnstone, Wellingborough.

Rogers, C.R. 1951: *Client Centred Therapy*. Constable, London.

Rogers, C.R. 1967: *On Becoming a Person*. Constable, London.

Rowe, D. 1990: Introduction. In Masson, J. (ed.), *Against Therapy*. Fontana, London.

Schulman, E.D. 1982: *Intervention in Human Services: A Guide to Skills and Knowledge*, 3rd edn. C.V. Mosby, St Louis, MO.

Sparkes, A.W. 1991: *Talking Philosophy: A Workbook*. Routledge, London.

Stewart, I. 1992: Risky Business. In Fifield, R. (ed.), *The New Scientist Inside Science: The Guide to Science Today*. Penguin, Harmondsworth, 329–42.

Stewart, W. 1983: *Counselling in Nursing: A Problem Solving Approach*. Harper & Row, London.

Stuart-Hamilton, I. 1994: *The Psychology of Ageing: An Introduction*, 2nd edn. Jessica Kingsley, London.

Thompson, I.E., Melia, K.M. and Boyd, K.M. 1988: *Nursing Ethics*. Churchill Livingstone, Edinburgh.

Tschudin, V. 1993: *Ethics: Aspects of Nursing Care*. Scutari, London.

Turner, B.S. 1986: *Medical Power and Social Knowledge*. Sage, London.

UKCC 1992: *Code of Professional Conduct*. United Kingdom Central Council for Nursing, Midwifery and Health Visiting, London.

UKCC 1996: *Guidelines for Professional Practice*. United Kingdom Central Council for Nursing, Midwifery and Health Visiting, London.

Walsh, M. and Ford, P. 1989: *Nursing Rituals: Research and Rational Action*. Butterworth-Heinemann, Oxford.

Woolf, F., Marsnik, N., Tacey, W. and Nichols, R. 1983: *Perceptive Listening*. Holt, Rinehart & Winston, New York.

Zeldin, T. 1994: *An Intimate History of Humanity*. Sinclair-Stevenson, London.

BIBLIOGRAPHY

Adler, R. and Rodman, G. 1988: *Understanding Human Communication*, 3rd edn. Holt, Rinehart & Winston, New York.

Adler, R.B., Rosenfield, L.B. and Towne, N. 1983: *Interplay: The Process of Interpersonal Communication*. Holt, Rinehart & Winston, London.

Adler, R.B. and Towne, N. 1984: *Looking Out/Looking In: Interpersonal Communication*. Holt, Rinehart & Winston, London.

Ajzen, I. 1988: *Attitudes, Personality and Behaviour*. Open University Press, Milton Keynes.

Allan, J. 1989: *How to Develop Your Personal Management Skills*. Kogan Page, London.

Argyle, M. (ed.) 1981: *Social Skills and Health*. Methuen, London.

Argyle, M. 1983: *The Psychology of Interpersonal Behaviour*: 4th Edition: Penguin, Harmondsworth.

Argyris, C. 1982: *Reasoning, Learning and Action*. Jossey Bass, San Francisco.

Argyris, C. and Schon, D. 1974: *Theory in Practice: Increasing Professional Effectiveness*. Jossey Bass, San Francisco.

Arnold, E. and Boggs, K. 1989: *Interpersonal Relationships: Professional Communication Skills for Nurses*. Saunders, Philadelphia.

Arnold, M.B. 1984: *Memory and the Brain*. Lawrence Erlbaum Associates, Hillsdale, NJ.

Aroskar, M.A. 1980a: Anatomy of an ethical dilemma: the theory, the practice. *American Journal of Nursing*. **80**(4), 658–63.

Aroskar, M.A. 1980b: Ethics of nurse–patient relationships. *Nurse Educator*. **5**(4), 18–20.

Baly, M. 1983: Based on trust. *Nursing Mirror*. **156**(12), 33–4.

Baly, M. 1984: *Professional Responsibility*. 2nd edn. Wiley, Chichester.

Barker, P. 1989: Reflections on the philosophy of caring in mental health. *International Journal of Nursing Studies*, **26**(2), 131–41.

Barnes, H.E. 1967: *An Existential Ethics*. Knopf, New York.

Barnes, R.D., Ickes, W.J. and Kidd, R.F. 1979: Effects of the perceived intentionality and stability of another's dependency on helping behaviour. *Personality and Social Psychology Bulletin* **5**, 367–72.

Baron, R.A. and Byrne, D. 1987: *Social Psychology: Understanding Human Interaction*, 5th edn. Allyn & Bacon, Boston, MA.

Bartley, W.W. 1971: *Morality and Religion*. Macmillan, London.

Baruth, L.G. 1987: *An Introduction to the Counselling Profession*. Prentice-Hall, Englewood Cliffs, NJ.

Beardshaw, V. 1981: *Conscientious Objectors at Work*. Social Audit, London.

Beauchamp, T.L. and Walter, L. 1978: *Contemporary Issues in Bioethics*. Dickenson, Encino, CA.

Beck, C.M., Crittenden, B.S. and Sullivan, E.V. (eds) 1971: *Moral Education*. Toronto University Press, Toronto.

Benjamin, M. and Curtis, J. 1981: *Ethics in Nursing*. Oxford University Press, New York.

Benner, P. 1984: *From Novice to Expert: Excellence and Power in Clinical Nursing Practice*. Addison-Wesley, Menlo Park, CA.

Benner, P. and Wrubel, J. 1989: *The Primacy of Caring: Stress and Coping in Health and Illness*. Addison Wesley, Menlo Park, CA.

Berry, C. 1987: *The Rites of Life: Christians and Bio-Medical Decision Making*. Hodder & Stoughton, London.

Blackham, H.J. 1968: *Humanism*. Pelican, Harmondsworth.

Blomquist, C., Veatch, R.M. and Fenner, D. 1975: The teaching of medical ethics. *Journal of Medical Ethics* **1**(2), 96–103.

Bok, S. 1980: *Lying: Moral Choice in Public and Private Life*. Quartet, London.

Bolger, A.W. (ed.) 1982: *Counselling in Britain: A Reader*. Batsford Academic, London.

Boud, D., Keogh, R. and Walker, M. 1985: *Reflection: Turning Experience into Learning*. Kogan Page, London.

Boud, D.J. (ed.) 1981: *Developing Student Autonomy in Learning*. Kogan Page, London.

Boydel, E.M. and Fales, A.W. 1983: Reflective learning: key to learning from experience. *Journal of Humanistic Psychology*. **23**(2), 99–117.

Brazier, M. 1987: *Medicine, Patients and the Law*. Pelican, Harmondsworth.

British Medical Association (BMA) 1980: *Handbook of Medical Ethics*. BMA, London.

Broad, C.D. 1930: *Five Types of Ethical Theory*. Routledge & Kegan Paul, London.

Brocket, R. and Hiemstra, R. 1985: Bridging the theory-practice gap in self-directed learning. In Brookfield, S.D. (ed.), *Self-Directed Learning: From Theory to Practice*. New Directions for Continuing Education No. 25. Jossey Bass, San Francisco, CA.

Brody, J.K. 1988: Virtue ethics, caring and nursing. *Scholarly Inquiry for Nursing Practice: An International Journal* **2**(2), 87–96.

Brookfield, S.D. 1987: *Developing Critical Thinkers: Challenging Adults to Explore Alternative Ways of Thinking and Acting*. Open University Press, Milton Keynes.

Brown, S.D. and Lent, R.W. (eds) 1984: *Handbook of Counselling Psychology*. Wiley, Chichester.

Calnan, J. 1983: *Talking with Patients*. Heinemann, London.

Campbell, A.V. 1981: *Rediscovering Pastoral Care*. Darton, Longman & Todd, London.

Campbell, A.V. 1984b: *Moral Dilemmas in Medicine*, 3rd edn. Churchill Livingstone, Edinburgh.

Campbell, A. 1985: *Paid to Care: The Limits of Professionalism in Pastoral Care*. SPCK, London.

Campbell, A.V. and Higgs, R. 1982: *In that Case*. Darton, Longman & Todd, London.

Carper, B.A. 1979: The ethics of caring. *Advances in Nursing Science* **1**(3), 11–19.

Carson B.V. 1989: *Spiritual Dimensions of Nursing Practice*. W.B. Saunders, Philadelphia.

Cash, K. 1990: Nursing models and the idea of nursing. *International Journal of Nursing Studies* **27**(3), 249–56.

Chapman, C.M. 1977: Concepts of professionalism. *Journal of Advanced Nursing* **2**, 51–5.

Claxton, G. 1984: *Live and Learn: An Introduction to the Psychology of Growth and Change in Everyday Life*. Harper & Row, London.

Clay, T. 1987: *Nurses: Power and Politics*. Heinemann, London.

Committee of Enquiry into Human Fertilisation and Embryology 1984: The Warnock Report. HMSO, London.

Cook, J. 1987: *Whose Health is it Anyway?* New English Library, Sevenoaks, Kent.

Dalley, G. 1988: *Ideologies of Caring: Rethinking Community and Collectivism*. Macmillan, London.

Daniels, V. and Horowitz, L.J. 1984: *Being and Caring: A Psychology for Living*, 2nd edn. Mayfield, Mountain View, CA.

Davis, A.J. and Aroskar, M.A. 1983: *Ethical Dilemmas and Nursing Practice*. Appleton-Century-Crofts, Norwalk, CT.

Davis, C.M. 1981: Affective education for the health professions. *Physical Therapy* **61**(11), 1587–93.

Davis, H. and Fallowfield, L. (eds). 1991: *Counselling and Communication in Health Care*. Wiley, Chichester.

de Bono, E. 1982: *de Bono's Thinking Course*. BBC, London.

De Vito, J.A. 1986: *The Interpersonal Communication Book*, 4th edn. Harper & Row, New York.

Dixon, D.N. and Glover, J.A. 1984: *Counselling: A Problem Solving Approach*. Wiley, Chichester.

Downie, R.S. and Calman, K.C. 1987: *Healthy Respect: Ethics in Health Care*. Faber & Faber, London.

Doxiadis, S. (ed.) 1987: *Ethical Dilemmas in Health Promotion*. Wiley, Chichester.

Dryden, W., Charles-Edwards, D. and Woolfe, R. 1989: *Handbook of Counselling in Britain*. Tavistock/Routledge, London.

Duncan, A.S., Dunstan, G.R. and Welbourne, R.B. 1981: *Dictionary of Medical Ethics*, 2nd edn. Darton, Longman & Todd, London.

Dunlop, M.J. 1986: Is a science of caring possible? *Journal of Advanced Nursing*, **11**, 661–70.

Dunstan, G.R. 1974: *The Artifice of Ethics*. SCM, London.

Dunstan, G.R. and Seller, M.J. (eds) 1983: *Consent in Medicine*. King Edward's Hospital Fund, London.

Durkheim, E. 1961: *Moral Education*. The Free Press, Glencoe, NY.

Ededel, A. 1955: *Ethical Judgement*. The Free Press, Glencoe, NY.

Evans, D. (ed.) 1990: *Why Should We Care?* Macmillan, London.

Ferguson, M. and Turner, V. 1976: The dilemma of professionalism and nursing organisation. *Nursing Mirror*, 16th December.

Fernando, S. 1990: *Mental Health, Race and Culture*. Macmillan, London.

Ferruci, P. 1982: *What We May Be*. Turnstone Press, Wellingborough.

Field, D. 1984: 'We didn't want him to die on his own' – nurses' accounts of nursing dying patients. *Journal of Advanced Nursing* **9**, 59–70.

Foggo-Pays, E. 1983: *An Introductory Guide to Counselling*. Ravenswood, Beckenham.

Forrest, D. 1989: The experience of caring. *Journal of Advanced Nursing* **14**, 815–23.

Frankena, W.K. 1973: *Ethics*. Prentice-Hall, Englewood Cliffs, NJ.

Frankl, V.E. 1978: *The Unheard Cry for Meaning*. Simon & Schuster, New York.

Fromm, E. 1976: *To Have or To Be?* Abacus, London.

Gardner, R.F.R. 1977: *By What Standard?* Christian Medical Federation , London.

General Medical Council (GMC) 1983: *Professional Conduct and Discipline; Fitness to Practice*. GMC, London.

Gibbs, G. 1981: *Teaching Students To Learn*. Open University Press, Milton Keynes.

Gibson, R.L. and Mitchell, M.H. 1986: *Introduction to Counselling and Guidance*. Collier Macmillan, London.

Glennerster, H. and Owens, P. 1990: *Nursing in Conflict*. Macmillan, London.

Goffman, I. 1971: *The Presentation of Self in Everyday Life*. Penguin, Harmondsworth.

Hall, J. 1990: Towards a psychology of caring. *British Journal of Clinical Psychology*, **29**, 129–44.

Halmos, P. 1965: *The Faith of the Counsellors*. Constable, London.

Hargie, O. (ed.) 1987: *A Handbook of Communication Skills*. Croom Helm, London.

Haring, B. 1974: *Medical Ethics*. St Paul Publications, Slough.

Harmin, M., Kirschenbaum, H. and Simon, S. 1973: *Clarifying Values Through Subject Matter*. Winston Press, Minneapolis.

Harris, J. 1986: *The Value of Life: An Introduction to Medical Ethics*. Routledge & Kegan Paul, London.

Harrison, L.L. 1990: Maintaining the ethic of caring in nursing. *Journal of Advanced Nursing* **15**, 125–7.

Hawkins, P. and Shohet, R. 1989: *Supervision and the Helping Professions*. Open University Press, Milton Keynes.

Heywood-Jones, I. 1990: *The Nurse's Code: A Practical Approach to the Code of Professional Conduct*. Macmillan, London.

Hirst, P.H. 1974: *Moral Education in a Secular Society*. University of London Press, London.

Howard, G.S., Nance, D.W. and Meyers, P. 1987: *Adaptive Counselling and Therapy: A Systematic Approach to Selecting Effective Treatments*. Jossey Bass, San Francisco, CA.

Hudson, W.D. 1970: *Modern Moral Philosophy*. Macmillan, London.

Hume, D. 1777: *Enquiry Concerning the Principles of Morals*. Edited by L.A. Selby-Bigge, 1902. Clarendon Press, Oxford.

Hurding, R.F. 1985: *Roots and Shoots: A Guide to Counselling and Psychotherapy*. Hodder & Stoughton, London.

Hyland, M. and Frapwell, C. 1986: Professional standards: rough justice. *Nursing Times* **82**(41), 32.

Illich, I. 1975: *Medical Nemesis: The Expropriation of Health*. Calder & Boyars, London.

International Council of Nurses (ICN) 1973: *Code of Nursing Ethics*. ICN, Geneva.

Ivey, A.E. 1987: *Counselling and Psychotherapy: Skills, Theories and Practice*. Prentice-Hall International, London.

Jackson, D.M. 1972: *Professional Ethics: Who Makes the Rules?* C.M.F. Publications, London.

Jarvis, P. 1983: Religiosity: a theoretical analysis of the human response to the problem of meaning. *Institute for the Study of Worship and Religious Architecture, Research Bulletin*, 51–66.

Jarvis, P. 1987: Meaningful and meaningless experience: towards an understanding of learning from life. *Adult Education Quarterly*, **37**, 3.

Jupe, M. 1987: Ethics and nursing practice. *Senior Nurse* **7**(3), 49–51.

Kemp, J. 1970: *Ethical Naturalism*. Macmillan, London.

Kennedy, E. 1979: *On Becoming a Counsellor*. Gill & Macmillan, London.

Kennedy, I. 1981: *Unmasking Medicine*. Allen & Unwin, London.

Kirschenbaum, H. 1977: *Advanced Values Clarification*. University Associates, La Jolla, CA.

Kleinig, J. 1985: *Ethical Issues in Psychosurgery*. Allen & Unwin, London.

Kleinman, A. 1988: *The Illness Narratives: Suffering, Healing and the Human Condition*. Basic Books, New York.

Knight, M. and Field, D. 1981: Silent conspiracy: coping with dying cancer patients on acute surgical wards. *Journal of Advanced Nursing* **6**, 221–9.

Levine, M. 1977: Ethics: nursing ethics and the ethical nurse. *American Journal of Nursing* **77**(5), 845–9.

Lewin, K. 1952: *Field Theory and Social Change*. Tavistock, London.

Lorber, J. 1975: Good patients and problem patients: conformity and deviance in a general hospital. *Journal of Health and Social Behaviour* **16**(2), 213–25.

Meyers, D.W. 1970: *The Human Body and the Law*. Edinburgh University Press, Edinburgh.

Mill, J.S. 1910: *Utilitarianism, Liberty and Representative Government*. Dent, London.

Moore, D. 1987: The buck stops with you. *Nursing Times* **83**(39), 54–6.

Moore, G.E. 1903: *Principia Ethica*. Cambridge University Press, Cambridge.

Morris, C. 1956: *Varieties of Human Value*. University of Chicago Press, Chicago.

Morrison, P. 1989: Nursing and caring: a personal construct theory study of some nurses' self-perceptions. *Journal of Advanced Nursing* **14**, 421–6.

Morrison, P. 1991: The caring attitude in nursing practice: a repertory grid study of trained nurses' perceptions. *Nurse Education Today* **11**, 3–12.

Morrison, P. and Burnard, P. 1991: *Caring and Communicating: The Interpersonal Relationship in Nursing*. Macmillan, London.

Munro, A., Manthei, B. and Small, J. 1988: *Counselling: The Skills of Problem-Solving*. Routledge, London.

Murgatroyd, S. 1986: *Counselling and Helping*. British Psychological Society & Methuen, London.

Murgatroyd, S. and Woolfe, R. 1982: *Coping with Crisis – Understanding and Helping Persons in Need*. Harper & Row, London.

Neuberger, J. 1987: *Caring for People of Different Faiths*. Austin Cornish, London.

Niblett, W.R. 1963: *Moral Education in a Changing Society*. Faber & Faber, London.

Nightingale, F. 1974: *Notes on Nursing: What It Is and What It Is Not*, 2nd edn. Blackie, London.

Phillips, M. and Dawson, J. 1985: *Doctors' Dilemmas: Medical Ethics and Contemporary Science*. Harvester Press, Brighton, Sussex.

Porritt, L. 1990: *Interaction Strategies: An Introduction for Health Professionals*, 2nd edn. Churchill Livingstone, Edinburgh.

Pyne, R. 1980: *Professional Discipline in Nursing*. Blackwell, London.

Pyne, R. 1987: A professional duty to shout. *Nursing Times*. **83**(42), 30–1.

Ramsey, P. 1965: *Deeds and Rules in Christian Ethics*. Cambridge University Press, Cambridge.

Ramsey, P. 1970: *The Patient as Person: Explorations in Medical Ethics*. Yale University Press, New Haven, CT.

Ramsey, P. 1978: *Ethics at the Edges of Life: Medical and Legal Intersections*. Yale University Press, New Haven, CT.

Rankin-Box, D.F. 1987: *Complementary Health Therapies: A Guide for Nurses and the Caring Professions*. Chapman & Hall, London.

Royal College of Nursing (RCN) 1976: *Code of Professional Conduct – A Discussion Document*. RCN, London.

Royal College of Nursing (RCN) 1977: *Ethics Related to Research in Nursing*. RCN. London.

Royal College of Nursing (RCN) 1979: *Charter and Byelaws*. RCN, London.

Rumbold, G. 1986: *Ethics in Nursing Practice*. Ballière Tindall, London.

Russell, P. 1979: *The Brain Book*. Routledge & Kegan Paul, London.

Salvage, J. 1985: *The Politics of Nursing*. Heinemann, London.

Samarel, N. 1989: Caring for the living and the dying: a study of role transition. *International Journal of Nursing Studies* **26**(4), 313–26.

Sampson, C. 1982: *The Neglected Ethic: Religious and Cultural Factors in the Care of Patients*. McGraw Hill, London.

Sarason, S.B. 1985: *Caring and Compassion in Clinical Practice*. Jossey Bass, London.

Sartre, J-P. 1973: *Existentialism and Humanism*. Translated by P. Mairet. Methuen, London.

Scammell, B. 1990: *Communication Skills*. Macmillan, London.

Schrock, R. 1980: A question of honesty in nursing practice. *Journal of Advanced Nursing* **5**(2), 135–48.

Scorer, G. and Wing, A. (eds) 1979: *Decision Making in Medicine: The Practice of its Ethics*. Edward Arnold, London.

Scott, R. 1981: *The Body as Property*. Viking Press, London.

Sieghart, P. 1985: Professions as the conscience of society. *Journal of Medical Ethics* **11**(3), 117–22

Simmons, D. 1982: *Personal Valuing: An Introduction*. Helson Hall, Chicago.

Simon, S.B., Howe, L.W. and Kirschenbaum, H. 1978: *Values Clarification: A Handbook of Practical Strategies for Teachers and Students*. A. and W. Visual Library, New York.

Strauss, A. 1978: *Negotiations: Varieties, Contexts and Social Order*. Jossey Bass, San Francisco, California.

Styles, M.M. 1982: *On Nursing: Towards A New Endowment*. C.V. Mosby: St Louis, MO.

Thiroux, J.P. 1980: Ethics, Theory and Practice, 2nd edn. Glencoe Publishing, Encino, CA.

Thompson, I.A., Melia, K. and Boyd, K. 1983: *Nursing Ethics*. Churchill Livingstone, Edinburgh.

Thompson, I.E. *et al.* 1981: Research Ethical Committees in Scotland. *British Medical Journal* **282**, 718–20.

Tshudin, V. and Schober, J. 1990: *Managing Yourself*. Macmillan, London.

UKCC 1984: *Code of Professional Conduct*. United Kingdom Central Council for Nursing, Midwifery and Health Visiting, London.

Van Hooft, S. 1987: Caring and professional commitment. *The Australian Journal of Advanced Nursing* **4**(4), 29–38.

Veatch, R.M. 1977: *Case Studies in Medical Ethics*. Harvard University Press, Cambridge, MA.

Warnock, M. 1970: *Existentialism*. Oxford University Press, London.

Watkins, J. 1978: *The Therapeutic Self*. Human Science Press, New York.

Watson, J. 1979: *Nursing: The Philosophy and Science of Caring*. Little, Brown, New York.

Watson, J. 1985: *Nursing: Human Science and Human Care: A Theory of Nursing*. Appleton-Century-Crofts, Norwalk, CT.

White, R. 1985: *Political Issues in Nursing*. Wiley, Chichester.

Williams, B. 1976: *Morality: An Introduction to Ethics*. Cambridge University Press, Cambridge.

Wright, D. 1971: *The Psychology of Moral Behaviour*. Penguin, Harmondsworth.

Young, A.P. 1981: *Legal Problems in Nursing Practice*. Harper & Row, London.

INDEX